Dilemmas and Decision Making in Cancer Care

This book presents realistic cancer-related clinical dilemmas and provides guidance on how to assess options and make ethical decisions.

The provided case studies explore how decisions are made in ethically and sometimes morally challenging situations in practice. Approaches to care delivery focus on the perspective of the individual in terms of their practical, social, psychological, and emotional needs. Considerations are integrated with a range of solutions-focused perspectives to allow readers to discuss clinical dilemmas in a safe space while applying and expanding their professional knowledge.

This book provides an invaluable resource for any healthcare student, clinical supervisor, academic educator, and anybody working within the cancer setting.

Julia Hubbard is a Professor of Clinical Health Education at the University of East Anglia (UEA) and a highly experienced academic, having worked in university-level healthcare education since 1993. During this time, she has been involved in curriculum development and course delivery across a range of healthcare professions, both at undergraduate and postgraduate levels, both nationally and internationally. Her current role as Department Head, Midwifery, Nursing and Nurse Apprenticeships, UEA, involves managing a large academic team who deliver a wide range of NMC-approved pre-registration programmes. She is also the Director of International Partnerships for the School of Health Sciences, UEA, supporting student travel abroad and fostering working and research partnerships with Health Science Schools across the globe.

Sarah Housden is an occupational therapist by background, now working as an Associate Professor in Health Sciences at the UEA. She has worked in healthcare and healthcare education for much of the past 30 years. This work has been in diverse contexts, including hospital, community, and social care settings, which have provided opportunities to meet and work alongside people living with a wide range of health conditions and social situations. Each of these people had a fascinating story to tell about their life experiences and achievements, often including journeys through cancer treatment and recovery. Sarah's passion as an educator is to promote healthcare provision which supports people to flourish, whatever their diagnosis or prognosis, so that patients' experiences in navigating choices and concerns around potential interventions and illness trajectories are as positive as possible.

Dilemmas and Decision Making
Series editor: Julia Hubbard

Dilemmas and Decision Making in Social Work
Abbi Jackson

Dilemmas and Decision Making in Residential Childcare
Abbi Jackson

Dilemmas and Decision Making in Midwifery
A Practice-Based Approach
Edited by Kenda Crozier, Julia Hubbard

Dilemmas and Decision Making in Dementia Care
Julia Hubbard, Sarah Housden

Dilemmas and Decision Making in Policing
Emma Spooner, Bob Cooper

Dilemmas and Decision Making in Nursing
A Practice-Based Approach
Edited by Julia Hubbard

Dilemmas and Decision Making in Cancer Care
A Practice-Based Approach
Edited by Julia Hubbard and Sarah Housden

For more information about this series please visit https://www.routledge.com/Dilemmas-and-Decision-Making/book-series/CRITDADM

Dilemmas and Decision Making in Cancer Care

A Practice-Based Approach

Edited by
Julia Hubbard
and Sarah Housden

Routledge
Taylor & Francis Group

LONDON AND NEW YORK

Designed cover image: Annette Fernando is an artist and illustrator whose practice spans drawing and film, drawing inspiration from her Sri Lankan, Italian, and French heritage. Based in London, her work has been exhibited in the UK, France, Spain, Sri Lanka, and Hong Kong. See annettefernando.carbonmade.com

First published 2026
by Routledge
4 Park Square, Milton Park, Abingdon, Oxon OX14 4RN

and by Routledge
605 Third Avenue, New York, NY 10158

Routledge is an imprint of the Taylor & Francis Group, an informa business

British Library Cataloguing-in-Publication Data
A catalogue record for this book is available from the British Library

ISBN: 978-1-041-09781-5 (hbk)
ISBN: 978-1-041-09780-8 (pbk)
ISBN: 978-1-003-65175-8 (ebk)

DOI: 10.4324/9781003651758

Typeset in Helvetica
by KnowledgeWorks Global Ltd.

Contents

About the contributors

Jennie Burch has been a nurse for over 30 years, predominantly in the field of colorectal nursing, where she discovered a love for writing and presenting on stoma care and is widely published in books and patient information material. Jennie has also worked in enhanced recovery after surgery (ERAS), helping patients recover faster and with fewer complications than with traditional care. The ERAS role included training colleagues in the UK and abroad on improving patient care. More recently, Jennie has been in a dedicated education role, developing post-registration colorectal study days, masterclasses, and university-accredited modules. Jennie currently teaches both pre-registration and post-registration nurses and nursing associates at Coventry University. Her PhD, from King's College London, focused on enhancing care for people after rectal cancer treatment by improving patient and colleague understandings of the support and management needed following these treatments.

Louise Grisedale is a pharmacist by background, an Associate Professor in pharmacology, and a Senior Fellow of the Higher Education Academy. She is the course director for the Independent Prescribing Programme and the MSc Advanced Professional Practice (APP) pathway at the University of East Anglia (UEA). Louise brings a wealth of experience in both clinical practice and academia, particularly in prescribing education and the development of advanced clinical practice. Louise's work focuses on delivering interactive and reflective teaching that supports healthcare professionals in developing safe, effective prescribing practices and enhancing patient-centred care.

Emma Harris is a registered adult nurse and has worked in acute medicine, urology, and general surgery before specialising in colorectal and upper gastroenterology care. Before joining the UEA, Emma held a specialist palliative care role in the National Health Service (NHS) and was project lead for Norfolk, implementing end-of-life education. Currently, Emma is an advanced communication skills facilitator for East Anglia, a role she has carried out for over 20 years. She also leads the UEA's Foundations of End-of-Life-Care teaching at the BSc and MSc levels.

Kirsty Henry is an Associate Professor in Health Sciences at the UEA, where she leads learning disability education practice. She is the module organiser for an MSc Advanced Learning Disability Practice module and for Complexity and Innovation in Nursing Practice in the pre-registration nursing BSc programme. Kirsty is a learning disability nurse with a clinical career focused on community healthcare for people with a learning disability and has a clinical and keen academic interest in reducing health inequalities as well as effective communication strategies.

Rebekah Hill is a registered adult nurse who has worked in the clinical fields of acute medicine, critical care, and gastroenterology/hepatology for many years. Rebekah now works as an Associate Professor and assessment lead in the School of Health Sciences at the UEA. She completed her PhD on the experience of living with hepatitis C and continues to work closely with gastroenterology and hepatology speciality groups.

Helen Humphrey is a lecturer in children and young people's nursing at the UEA. Helen's clinical background is varied and includes both acute and community paediatrics. Before joining UEA, Helen was a Clinical Nurse Specialist in Paediatric Palliative Care and Symptom Management, working with children, young people with life-threatening and life-limiting conditions, and their families. Helen teaches across both the BSc and MSc Nursing programmes and is a module organiser and practice education lead for Children and Young People's Nursing. Helen's particular areas of interest are communication skills around difficult conversations, the importance of developing professionally curious nurses, health inclusivity, and the integration of palliative care as a total and holistic approach to patient care and management.

Chrysi Leliopoulou is a mixed methods researcher with a special interest in evidence-based clinical practice, cancer care, clinical decision-making and physical examination competence, workforce development, affective well-being, and emotionality. She was sponsored as a research fellow role with the Marie Curie Research Centre and led research and teaching in advanced communication skills for senior cancer nurses funded by GlaxoSmithKline and accredited by the Royal College of Nursing. Chrysi has worked as a senior nurse in bone marrow transplant units at the Royal Free Hospital Foundation Trust and UCL Hospital Foundation Trust, and currently works as an Associate Professor at the UEA.

Paul Linsley has worked largely in acute and forensic mental health settings both as a clinician and as a manager. He is registered as a clinical specialist in acute psychiatry and is trained in Cognitive Behavioural Therapy, Coaching, and Reality Therapy. As an Associate Professor for the UEA, he teaches several courses, both single and joint honours undergraduate programmes, research Master's programmes and pre- and post-registration specialist mental health programmes. He supervises Doctoral students and sits on several special interest panels and committees relating to mental health.

Jayne Needham is an Associate Professor at the UEA and Lead Midwife for Education. She is an experienced lecturer and registered midwife, having qualified in 1988. She has expertise and research interests in high-dependency midwifery and critical care. Her doctoral studies were aligned with this area of midwifery. She has experience in curriculum development in the UK and India, and continues to collaborate with Indian colleagues in the education of the midwifery global workforce.

Christine Nightingale is a learning disability nurse by background and has worked across the NHS, commissioning, education, and higher education sectors, promoting equality, equity, and inclusion. Her research has focused on sexual health, health inequalities for people with learning disabilities, mental health, disabled staff working in post-16 education, and embedding equality and diversity into education. She is a nominated Fellow of the Royal Society of Arts and a Senior Fellow of the Higher Education Academy.

Marie O'Donovan is an experienced registered children's nurse with a Master's degree in Children's Advanced Practice from London South Bank University. With a rich and diverse career, she has dedicated many years to paediatric haematology, oncology, and bone marrow transplant. As a leukaemia clinical nurse specialist, she played a pivotal role in patient care, which later led her to an Advanced Nurse Practitioner position in paediatric haematology, oncology, and bone marrow transplant. Her extensive clinical background and expertise are now shared with the next generation of nurses through her role as a lecturer at the UEA. Marie is deeply passionate about teaching, with a focus on applied anatomy, physiology, and the integration of clinical cases into nursing education for both undergraduate and postgraduate students.

Simon Rose is a specialist paramedic in primary and urgent care, working in clinical areas such as the advanced practice team within the ambulance service. Now at the UEA, Simon is a lecturer on the BSc Paramedic Science programme and has contributed to a variety of postgraduate modules on the Advanced Professional Practice Masters. His current role as a Director of the School of Health Sciences involves him leading key strategic workstreams such as admissions, recruitment, and marketing for a wide range of healthcare professions.

Ruth Sanders is an Associate Professor at the UEA and a Senior Fellow of the Higher Education Academy. She is an experienced lecturer and registered midwife with research interests including advanced clinical practice in midwifery, decision-making and health communication, and research methods. Ruth is currently undertaking a Professional Doctorate in Health and Social Care focused on student's experiences of creative reflective practice and is a Professional Midwifery Advocate supporting students in the academic setting. She sits on the Royal College of Midwives Editorial Board, as well as contributing to the advisory panel in her role as an ambassador for Cavell, a charity supporting nursing and midwifery professionals. Ruth has been involved in the development of advancing clinical practice in midwifery nationally. She is a visiting tutor for King's College London and enjoys reviewing and writing for a range of midwifery journals.

Gabrielle Thorpe is a Professor of Professional Development in Health Sciences at the UEA. Gabby practised as a Colorectal and Stoma Care Specialist Nurse from 1997 to 2020. Since 2009, this was alongside her academic role, through which she has taught different aspects of colorectal surgery and stoma care at all academic levels and contributed to a wide body of research in this area. Her PhD, awarded in 2012, focused on the experience of living with a new stoma, focusing on changes in the relationship between body and self, created by stoma formation and how people with a stoma re-establish their sense of embodied self, following stoma formation. Over the past 25 years, Gabby has worked with many national organisations and charities, through which she has supported professional development for gastrointestinal nurses and sought to improve the lives of people with bowel disease. She was Chair of the Association of Coloproctology Nurses (2019–2023) and sits on the PPI and Research Grants Committees for Bowel Research UK.

Katherine Waterfall is a midwife by background, currently working as a Midwifery Lecturer at the UEA and undertaking her PhD at City St George's University of London. Katherine is passionate about Anti-Racism within healthcare education and decolonial pedagogical practice. Katherine is co-Chair of the UEA School of Health Sciences (HSC) Anti-Racism working group and leads on decolonising midwifery education at UEA. Katherine is also co-convenor of a national network of midwifery educators working on decolonial approaches to midwifery education. Katherine is an expert in the field of maternal care for women seeking sanctuary in the UK. Within this capacity, Katherine sits on the NHS Race and Health Observatory working group for Maternal and Neonatal Racial Inequalities, the Home Office sub-group for maternal health and Maternity Action's panel analysing the procedural fairness of NHS charging regulations.

Emma Watts trained as a learning disabilities registered nurse at the UEA in 2012. She took up her first qualified post as a renal nurse at the Norfolk and Norwich University Hospital in 2015, becoming dialysis trained in 2016. After six years as a ward nurse and deputy sister, she transitioned into the renal educator role where she works now, supporting staff and student nurses on placement. Emma's professional interests include teaching and participation in clinical treatments such as dialysis and plasmapheresis.

Introduction

Presented primarily from the perspective of the practitioner involved in providing care and support, each case study in this book provides opportunities to safely experience and discuss clinical dilemmas through cases which are true to life while being theoretically modelled, providing space to explore your personal values and beliefs. You will be able to relate your own practice to relevant theoretical models and concepts while applying and expanding your professional knowledge to promote your ongoing professional development.

Key themes running throughout the book are healthcare values, individual choice, challenges and opportunities, personalised care, quality of life, and living with and beyond a cancer diagnosis. The case studies in the chapters that follow explore how decisions are made in ethically and sometimes morally challenging situations in practice, enabling the reader to consider the effect of applying several approaches to care delivery. These approaches focus variously on the perspective of individuals in terms of their practical, social, psychological and emotional needs, as well as the viewpoints of others involved in the person's life and care.

Cancer will touch all of us in our lifetime, either as a personal diagnosis or by affecting someone we know or care for. Statistically, this paints the following picture:

- More than 900,000 cancer deaths within the next five years (Wedekind, 2024).

- Over three million people live with cancer in the UK. This figure is expected to rise to four million people by the end of 2030 and 5.3 million people by 2040 (Macmillian Cancer Support, 2024).

- Approximately 167,000 people die each year in the UK from cancer, averaging at least 460 deaths a day (Macmillian Cancer Support, 2024).

- The NHS diagnosed over 11,000 more cancers in 2022, reaching a record high with almost 950 diagnoses per day in England alone (NHS England, 2024).

These statistics highlight the significant impact of cancer in the UK and the potential ongoing challenges in cancer care and prevention. NHS England (2023) has introduced a new target called the Faster Diagnosis Standard. This relates to the percentage of patients who receive a diagnosis of cancer within 28 days. This will impact the number of referrals for cancer treatment and care. In addition, decisions made in practice may be influenced by the quality measures outlined by the Quality Surveillance Team.

In response to the above challenges, the content of this book is implicitly mapped to the Aspirant Cancer Career and Education Development Framework (ACCEND)

(NHS England, 2023) to enable you to understand the cancer journey from diagnosis to death, reflecting the part healthcare professionals play in this journey.

Section 1: Navigating the complexities of diagnosis and treatment

Chapters explore and build on competency around understandings of cancer diagnosis (Sylvia), breaking the diagnostic news to family (Sandra and Erica), decisions on whether to accept (Lily) or decline treatment (Ravi) and discussing dying and care planning with children and their families (Claire).

Section 2: Living well with cancer

For some individuals, cancer becomes a long-term condition which they need to learn to live with. The future could mean living with the long-lasting impact of treatment and changes to an individual's body image (Michelle and Antony); managing treatments, symptoms and pain (Paul and Priya); living with the fear that the cancer could return (Jack); or facing racial stigma during treatment (Aakifah).

Section 3: Towards the end of life

An individual reaching the end of their cancer journey will respond in unique ways. From recognising a life lived well (Garreth) to fear of dying (Becky and Will) and the complexities involved in supporting people to make decisions around the options for treatment and care at the end of life (Ben, Zach, and Sandy).

The model of decision making in the above scenarios reflects a partnership approach to cancer care, often described as 'person centred care,' the importance of which is highlighted throughout this book. Service providers within cancer care often face dilemmas in deciding whether to provide survival statistics, discuss life expectancy and poor diagnosis, or encourage hope while being mindful of a range of potential cultural and social barriers to communication.

The contributors' annotations in the margins of each case provide the opportunity to follow their thinking processes, as the presentation of the case studies mirrors the process of thinking aloud, thus enabling readers to unpack the elements of each situation and to develop a systematic and logical approach to decision making. The benefits of this approach include the opportunity to explore professional dilemmas which can be difficult to respond effectively when first coming across them in practice settings. This supports the acquisition of understanding and knowledge which will support your future decision making when working with people living with cancer.

How to use this book

This book can be read in several ways. You are invited to work through the case studies in the order of presentation or to dip in and out of the case studies as free-standing sources of information matched to your specific learning requirements at any time. Each case study starts with a fictitious but true-to-life clinical scenario told from the perspective of the healthcare professional. These scenarios provide an insight into the various aspects of cancer practice and simultaneously impart the professionals' underlying thinking and evidence-informed decision-making processes. Provided as 'shout outs' in the margins of the text, links are made with numerous approaches, values, models, and theories, which demonstrate how healthcare professionals make use of a wide range of tools and perspectives as part of appraising available options as robust clinical decisions are made in complex situations. These concepts are explained in more depth at the end of each scenario in a further information section.

The case studies also include the health professionals' reflections either in action (while it is happening) or on action (after the event), providing further insight into how clinical decisions must evolve based on the evidence available. A set of reflective questions then provides an opportunity for you to consider your own knowledge and learning, and how to apply these in practice settings. We hope that you find the questions stimulating and that you will take the opportunity to read further about the key areas of cancer practice.

In anticipation that you will want to relate your reading to your clinical practice, each case study provides some suggestions and resources to support further study. We would encourage you to work with either a peer or clinical supervisor to ensure you expose yourself to a variety of differing perspectives and analyse what you may, or may not, have done differently. By scrutinising and reflecting on day-to-day practice, you will develop your understanding of the importance of being able to justify, sometimes to multiple audiences, the thinking and rationale underpinning your professional judgements.

Use Diagram 0.1 to help you work through the case studies in a systematic and considered way.

Finally, try looking through alternative lenses for each case. Such lenses could include, for example, age, gender, ethnicity, culture, religion, disability, trauma, domestic abuse, relationships, sexual orientation, learning needs, poverty, stigma, mental or physical health needs, carer status, personality, needs or neglect, loss and grief, homelessness status, world view, or the views of other professionals (Jackson, 2021). Consider what lenses you habitually add, or could add, to each scenario.

My personal analysis

Review of the case study

Best practice standards

What are my initial reactions to the scenario?

What are the facts of the situation (e.g. history, signs and symptoms, test results)

What is the relevant guidance from my professional standards?

What is the context? (e.g. issues, people, values, culture)

Case study analysis

What are my legal and organisational obligations in the situation presented?

Which principles are relevant?

What is considered best practice? (e.g. clinical guidelines NICE, research evidence)

What actions would I take and why?

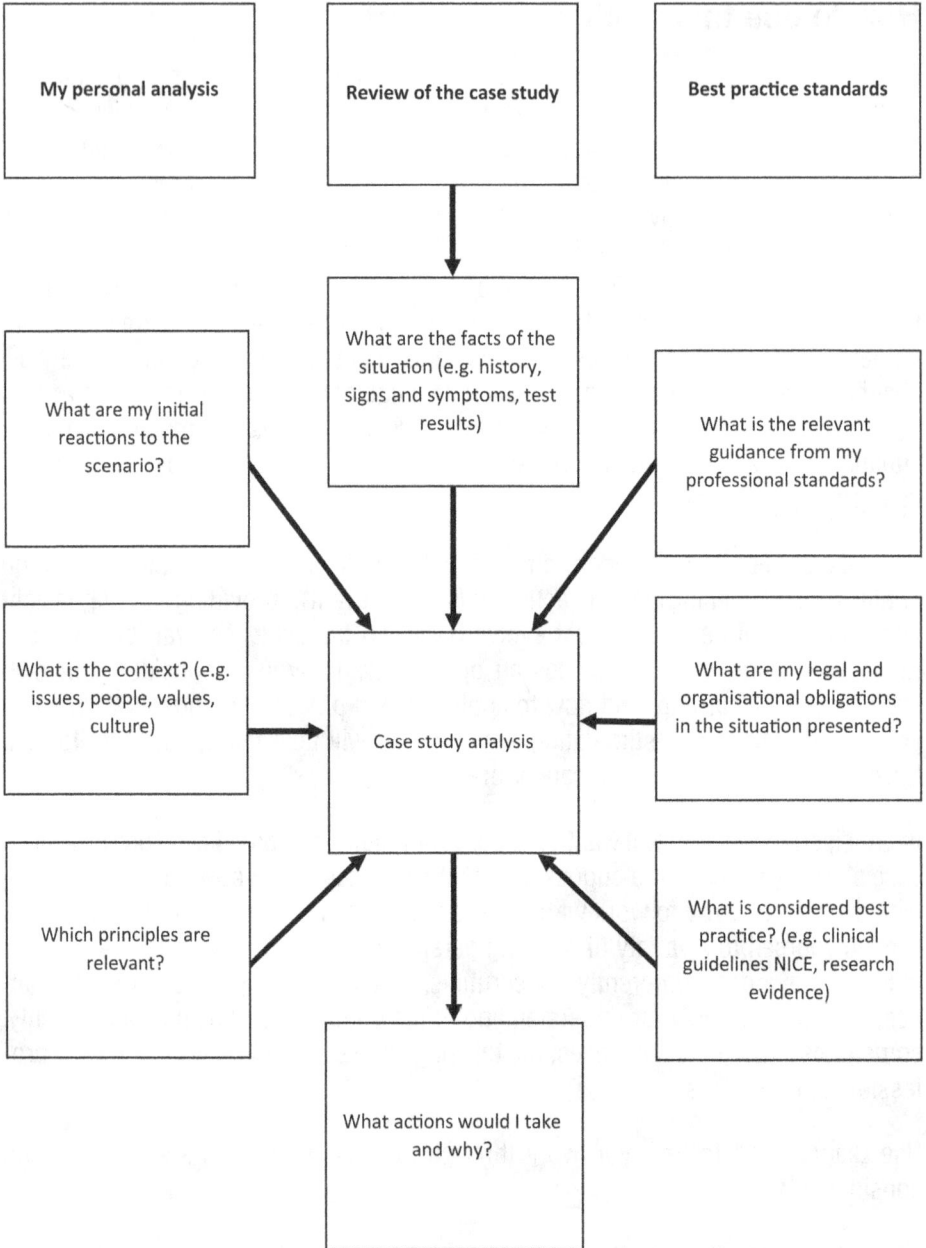

Diagram 0.1 An approach to working through the case studies.

Adapted with permission from Jackson (2021).

References

Jackson, A. (2021) *Dilemmas and Decision Making in Social Work*. St. Albans, Critical Publishing.

Macmillian Cancer Support (2024) *Statistical Fact Sheet*. Cancer statistics fact sheet | Macmillan Cancer Support (Accessed 24th February 2024).

NHS England (2023) *Aspirant Cancer Career and Education Development Framework*. https://www.hee.nhs.uk/our-work/cancer-diagnostics/aspirant-cancer-career-education-development-programme/accend-framework (Accessed 24th February 2025).

NHS England (2024) *NHS diagnoses thousands more cancers as cases rise by 5% NHS* England. NHS diagnoses thousands more cancers as cases rise by 5% (Accessed 24th February 2024). https://www.england.nhs.uk/2024/10/nhs-diagnoses-thousands-more-cancers-as-cases-rise-by-5/

Wedekind, S. (2024) *More than 900,000 cancer deaths predicted in the next 5 years*. https://news.cancerresearchuk.org/2024/09/09/more-than-900000-cancer-deaths-predicted-in-the-next-5-years/ (Accessed 24th February 2025).

Case study 1
Sylvia: beyond labels

Sarah Housden

Sylvia's referral

Working as a recently qualified occupational therapist in the oncology outpatient clinic, I find myself with diverse opportunities to undertake assessments and provide interventions, which, depending on prognosis, include supporting patients with equipment to help with self-care tasks, advising on ways to save their energy and combat fatigue during treatment, and exploring ways of maintaining or returning to paid work or other meaningful occupation. There are also opportunities to provide psycho-emotional interventions to support adjustment to changing levels of ability and disability, as well as sometimes working with individuals and their families as they explore more existential questions as part of preparing for their impending death.

THEORY: occupational meaning

APPROACH: whole person care

It is for the latter purpose that I assume Sylvia has been referred to me. She is a 79-year-old woman of African-Caribbean heritage who was diagnosed with early-stage vascular dementia a year ago and with stage 2 stomach cancer in the past three months. The referring clinician has said that she is not suitable for surgery due to what are described as complicating factors in her current situation, which affect her capacity to understand the instructions associated with following the post-surgery lifestyle and diet guidance. The referral suggests that the best course of action is psychosocial interventions to support the patient in understanding the diagnosis and prognosis, followed by discharge until such time as a more palliative approach might be required.

APPROACH: biomedicine

MODEL: stages of dementia

MODEL: family of dementias

THEORY: long-term management

My curiosity about Sylvia's perspective arises immediately as I wonder how she might be coping with a cancer diagnosis on top of the adjustments that are likely to have been

VALUE: curiosity

DOI: 10.4324/9781003651758-1

required due to cognitive changes occurring with her vascular dementia. I am interested to hear Sylvia's story and to establish the part she played in the decision not to pursue surgical treatment for stomach cancer. To gain a fuller picture of Sylvia's situation, there are a few questions I would like to ask her and clinicians who have assessed and supported her to this point.

Meeting Sylvia

I walk into the waiting room and call Sylvia's name. Two sprightly older women stand up, along with a man I presume to be the partner of one of them.

'That's us,' they say in unison, all three stepping forward with big smiles on their faces.

'Ah, and which one of you is Sylvia?' I ask, returning the smile.

'That'll be me' says the shorter of the two women. 'And this is my husband Cedric and my younger sister Gloria.'

'Hello, my name is Rosie, and I'll be seeing you today,' I say, while simultaneously thinking about the hospital rules which advise that only one relative or other carer is permitted to join patients in need of support while attending appointments. I quickly weigh up some potential reasons for all three of them needing to be here. The waiting room

is not the place for sharing personal support needs, so I ask Sylvia whether she would like both Gloria and Cedric to come into the clinic room with her.

'Oh yes, yes please, that's just what I need,' replies Sylvia, with a smile, while Gloria and Cedric enthusiastically nod their agreement.

I lead them down the short corridor and, at the door of my allocated clinic room, invite them in. Due to all three of the available chairs being taken, I draw up a perching stool which is sitting in the corner, and after checking some key personal details with Sylvia, I begin by explaining the purpose of the appointment.

VALUE: communication

'So, first things first, Sylvia. I'm Rosie, and I'm an occupational therapist. I have been asked to see you by your consultant Mr Wilson, to see how we can best support you with your recent diagnosis. So today we'll just run through how things are with your health right now, how well you're coping with everyday tasks, and any feelings you'd like to discuss about what's happening. There will be time to ask as well as answer questions, and then we'll make a plan for going forward.' I speak at a moderately steady pace, slightly slower than usual because I'm mindful that Sylvia may have difficulty concentrating. I pause to check that she is following me. She has maintained eye contact and has a quizzical look on her face, alongside a slight smile.

APPROACH: explanation

THEORY: non-verbal communication

Taking her smile to indicate interest and understanding, I continue: 'It can be a difficult time, adjusting to a cancer diagnosis. I wonder whether you can tell me a bit about yourself and how your health is at the moment, to begin with.'

Sylvia continues to look at me with a slight smile and a quizzical facial expression but does not speak. I reflect on what I've said and realise that in attempting to orient Sylvia to how the appointment would proceed, I had probably provided too much information in one go. I make an inward note to talk about only one thing at a time and try again.

APPROACH: reflection on action

'Sylvia, how are you feeling about being here today?' I ask.

'I'm not sure,' she answers. 'I'm worried I'm going to be told bad news. I'm worried I might be dying. That's not news anyone wants to hear, is it Rosie?'

I notice that Sylvia remembers my name, suggesting her short-term memory for information is functional to some extent. Yet it seems as though she does not remember being told that her cancer is inoperable. I wonder to myself what Mr Wilson has or has not told her.

APPROACH: assessment by observation

MODEL: types of memory

VALUES: honesty

Gloria moves to put an arm around her older sister's shoulder. Cedric is the next to speak:

'We are quite uncertain about things,' he says, his tone full of sadness. 'Mr Wilson says Sylvia has cancer but can't have treatment and we don't understand why. My son looked up stage 2 stomach cancer on his computer and he says that the doctors should be able to do something to help – if only to give my wife another few good years on this earth with me.'

Internally, the alarm bells that started sounding quietly a few minutes ago are now ringing loud and clear. The first thing I need to do is to better understand Sylvia's perspective, find out about her home circumstances, and assess her daily functioning. Then I will take a look at what assessment has been made of her mental capacity. One thing at a time, I remind myself.

Sylvia's story

Sylvia's smile at first broadens and then diminishes as she begins to speak. 'I've never been unwell, my entire life, until I had the difficulty with organising cooking and household jobs. The doctor sent me to the Memory Clinic, even though my memory isn't much of a problem, and the doctor there said this difficulty organising was part of dementia'. I nod, showing my understanding and being keen to hear more from Sylvia.

A perplexed expression spreads over Sylvia's face as she tells me about feeling quite at ease with the diagnosis, although not really understanding it. She continues: 'It was just two months after that when I started getting these pains in my tummy so went back to the doctor to get help with that.' I keep my gaze steady and my face as calm as possible as Sylvia tells me that she was told that the abdominal pain and what felt like persistent indigestion were probably stress-related following her dementia diagnosis.

'We wouldn't let it rest at that though,' says Gloria, looking directly at Sylvia. 'She was in so much pain, and she'd never been one to be off her food, but she lost her appetite over the next few weeks. So, we went back to the doctor together – me, Sylvia and Cedric, and we insisted on a referral to the hospital. We wouldn't take no for an answer.'

'That's how we first came to be here in this clinic last month,' Cedric explains. 'But the thing I don't understand – none of us understand – is why, when they know now that Sylvia has cancer, they aren't treating her for it as soon as possible. Can you tell us, Rosie?'

Assessing Sylvia

I spend over an hour with Sylvia, Gloria, and Cedric. At the end of the hour, I have a good picture of how supportive of each other they and the wider family are. Gloria and Cedric are providing regular guidance with tasks which require planning and organisation, as this is a key area of cognitive functioning which is impaired for Sylvia. However, her memory for both autobiographical and factual information from the recent past appears to be largely intact, demonstrated by her having a good understanding of both her diagnoses and being able to follow instructions throughout a structured occupational therapy assessment.

THEORY: family carers

THEORY: cognitive impairment

APPROACH: strengths-based practice

MODEL: validated assessments

What she and her family do not understand is why the stomach cancer is not being treated. I do not understand either, although I suspect that it may have something to do with assumptions being made about her mental capacity and ability to care for herself following surgery. Following my assessment of her ability to carry out activities of daily living, as well as to follow instructions, my initial thought is that Sylvia may be being stereotyped and discriminated against due to her age and dementia diagnosis and possibly being treated according to the labels instead of as an individual. I am keen that she should be assessed as having a unique profile of strengths and limitations, as well as a lifetime's experience of managing in difficult situations.

THEORY: avoiding assumptions

VALUE: self-awareness

THEORY: stereotyping

VALUE: non-discriminatory practice

THEORY: labelling

THEORY: unconscious bias

APPROACH: person-centred practice

APPROACH: valuing experience

I want to talk to Mr Wilson to ascertain whether my suspicions have any basis in fact. I do not want to be confrontational, but I am curious about how Sylvia has been assessed and

APPROACH: advocacy

VALUE: collaboration

whether some misunderstandings or inaccurate judgements may have been made about her abilities due to her age and dementia diagnosis.

APPROACH: clinical supervision

First, though, I need to pass this on to my clinical supervisor, with whom I arrange a meeting for the following day. I do not want to waste time waiting to talk this through. Every day that passes, as I see it, will change Sylvia's prognosis and her suitability for surgery.

A meeting with my clinical supervisor

Jennifer looks up, smiles, and beckons me to come in and sit down when I knock on the door to her office. It cannot be easy for Mr Wilson, I think to myself, having to give so many people the news about their diagnosis – some of whom will not have long to live. He must see a lot of shocked reactions, a lot of tears, and even more putting on of brave faces.

APPROACH: empathy

THEORY: practitioner resilience

I waste no time in getting to the point with Jennifer: 'I had a patient in Mr Wilson's clinic yesterday. She has vascular dementia and has more recently been diagnosed with stomach cancer. I carried out several assessments to establish her level of functioning, as is my usual approach with patients in this clinic, and she seems to be doing well for someone with dementia.' I pause to see if she is following me, and that, in my anxiety to be an advocate and argue Sylvia's case, I am explaining clearly enough.

APPROACH: communication with colleagues

'She has been told that due to complications she will not be having surgery for her Stage 2 stomach cancer,' I say, waiting for a response from Jennifer.

'What complications are they?' she asks, seeking to better understand Sylvia's situation. 'If the cancer is inoperable for whatever reason, surely she can be offered alternative non-invasive treatments?'. This is something I had been wondering too. I explain to her my concerns about potential discrimination against an older person and the complicating factor of perceptions of dementia in society.

APPROACH: questioning in communication

THEORY: ageism

THEORY: social stigma of dementia

Jennifer and I talk through the assessments I have carried out, and she confirms that these are appropriate, but then states without hesitation that this does not mean that I have as full a picture of Sylvia's situation and of her cancer as Mr Wilson does. Jennifer looks me directly in the eyes and, with a calm, steady tone of voice, says:

VALUE: objectivity

'Rosie, think about the broader picture. It is possible that you are jumping to conclusions about other people making assumptions, without making sure of the full facts first. You run the risk of making false accusations about a senior doctor, and therefore a fool of yourself, when ultimately you have no evidence of wrongdoing on Mr Wilson's or anyone else's part. I think you need to tread cautiously. Let's talk through all we know again, but this time, let's start with the assumption that Mr Wilson and his team truly are acting in Sylvia's best interests.'

THEORY: rank dynamics

I am hesitant to consider other alternatives but I realise that critical thinking and reflection are essential skills which I need to develop. Jennifer supports me as I begin to talk through alternative ways of seeing this scenario.

APPROACH: reflective practice

THEORY: perspectives on reality

'If Sylvia were to have this surgery, what are the risks associated with a lengthy anaesthetic when she already has impaired cognitive functioning? I haven't really considered that. Then there's the risks associated with spending time in an unfamiliar environment during post-operative recovery, which would increase the chances of developing delirium, which are already higher in people living with dementia. I also need to think through the longer term – after the immediate post-operative recovery. Sylvia will permanently need to eat much smaller meals than she is used to and if her memory becomes more impaired, she may not understand the need for this. And of course, what sort of quality of life are we going to be able to support for Sylvia in the longer term, as her dementia will continue to progress and ultimately lead to increased disorientation, affecting every part of her life until ultimately she dies with more advanced dementia if not of the complications of the dementia itself.

APPROACH: professional decision-making

THEORY: quality of life in dementia

THEORY: domains of dementia

THEORY: illness trajectories

Jennifer sits back and asks me what I think. I answer with as much assurance as I had held at the start of this meeting, but now with a different focus.

'Jennifer, thanks for helping me see this more clearly. The poor practice that appears to have been made, if any, is in not involving Sylvia and her family in the decision-making process. After all, she may decide for herself that she would rather have a better quality of life for a shorter amount of time.'

'Absolutely. Or she may decide that she wants the surgery if she is medically fit to have it. We don't know. And neither do we know whether Mr Wilson has already considered all these things and discussed them with Sylvia and her family. Receiving a diagnosis of cancer is a time of such heightened emotion for anyone, never mind for a person living with dementia. Maybe we should ask Mr Wilson for some further details about what he knows of Sylvia's case and wider circumstances. Let's not go making any accusations but instead act with a healthy curiosity to find out more.'

I feel rather embarrassed about my initial approach and the assumptions I made. At the same time, I am grateful for Jennifer's supportive approach in helping me to take a step back and reflect on this.

'What should I do now?' I ask.

'What would you like to do?' replies Jennifer, modelling that shared decision-making process that we've just been talking about.

'I think I'd like to talk with Mr Wilson, and share my findings from assessments, while at the same time asking him for a fuller picture of what he has discussed with Sylvia and her family.' I answer.

'Great,' says Jennifer. 'Let's do that next week at the multi-disciplinary team meeting before Mr Wilson's next clinic. It will help us both if we get a fuller picture of the decision-making process.'

Jennifer smiles as I get up to leave her office. As I open the door, her parting words resonate strongly with me: 'Every day is a learning day Rosie, and every day that we do our best for our patients is a good day at work. Maintain a curious mind, keep asking questions and avoid jumping to conclusions and your skills and confidence will grow as a colleague and as a therapist.'

Reflections

There is no absolute clarity in this scenario about whether decisions have been made in a way that is discriminatory or based on stereotypical views of people living with dementia, but research evidence suggests that healthcare professionals and organisations need to be more aware that older people are liable to age-related prejudice and stereo-typing processes within healthcare settings (Swift et al., 2016). Discriminatory attitudes may be more prevalent in acute healthcare settings, where the swift processing of patients is encouraged. Older people, especially those with more complex needs, who require longer to recover from surgery and may also need rehabilitation, can be perceived as problematic within a system aiming for early discharges (Kydd and Fleming, 2015). Add to this the potential for dis-crimination based on Sylvia's dementia diagnosis, and it is clear why Rosie holds some concerns about whether Sylvia has been properly informed and consulted about options for treatment. Indeed, Farhana et al. (2023) highlight that the stigmatising way in which stereotypes of dementia are constructed leads to family caregivers and people with dementia alike being treated poorly within health services. Therefore, reflection upon the assumptions we make and awareness of potential unconscious biases are central to being able to make fair and equitable professional decisions in healthcare settings.

At the heart of Sylvia's case is the need to take a person-centred approach to treatment planning and patient care (McCormack et al., 2021). Whatever our views about the person's likelihood of achieving or maintaining quality of life, they (and their family, where consent is given for this) should have a role in decision-making processes, at least to the degree of feeling involved and being able to understand the reasons behind decisions made, even when not agreeing with these.

A paternalistic approach, where decisions are made in what the medical or healthcare team consider to be the best interests of a vulnerable person, is still seen at times in settings where a more biomedical approach is taken (Farre and Rapley, 2017). This can lead to a prioritisation of the task (the delivery of cancer treatments) taking precedence over the person, and thus to a disempowering approach to the delivery of cancer services. Following the guidance for making assessments of an individual's capacity in line with the principles of the Mental Capacity Act (2005) helps to avoid making wrong assumptions about an individual's ability to make decisions at any time on any specific matter, regardless of diagnosis. It is also essential that, where a person is assessed as not having the capacity to make a specific decision at a specific time, they are still involved, communicated with, and asked for their views. Where available, information on any views expressed in the past about the acceptability of different cancer treatments can also be taken into consideration.

These matters also highlight the importance of effective and inclusive communication, as well as Advanced Care Planning, Lasting Power of Attorney, and Advance Decisions to Refuse Treatment. Further information on legal aspects of supporting decision-making with a person living with dementia, as relevant to a UK setting, can be found on the Dementia UK (2022) and Alzheimer's Society (2024) websites (see references).

Questions for reflection and discussion

Explore the key issues raised in the above scenario as you answer the following six questions:

1. What features of the individual are taken into account when making decisions about the provision of lifesaving and life-prolonging treatments within a service setting with which you are familiar?

2. Identify ways in which other professionals with specialist expertise can be involved in supporting patients living with dementia to contribute to decision-making processes around their treatments and aftercare.

3. Describe the potential risks and benefits associated with shared decision-making and involving patients with limited or impaired cognition in decision-making.

4. Identify a variety of risks associated with making assumptions and jumping to conclusions in relation to both patients and colleagues within cancer care settings.

5. Identify how you would approach a similar situation to that experienced by Rosie in a way which enhances collaborative working between professionals to the benefit of patients.

6. In the light of Rosie's evolving thought processes within this scenario, explore the value that structured approaches to clinical supervision and reflective practice can bring to providing person-centred cancer services.

Further reading

Braveman, B. and Newman, R. (2020) *Cancer and Occupational Therapy: Enabling Performance and Participation Across the Lifespan*, Bethesda, MD: AOTA.

Housden, S. (author) and Hubbard, J. (editor) (2023) *Dilemmas and Decision Making in Dementia Care*, St Albans: Critical Publishing.

Maclean, F., Warren, A. and Westcott, L. (2022) *Occupational Therapy and Dementia: Promoting Inclusion, Rights and Opportunities for People Living with Dementia*, London: Jessica Kingsley Publishers.

Scaife, J. (2019) *Supervision in Clinical Practice: A Practitioner's Guide*, London: Routledge.

Schell, B. and Schell, J. (2023) *Clinical and Professional Reasoning in Occupational Therapy*, Alphen aan den Rijn: Wolters Kluwer Health.

Further information

VALUES

Caring involves practitioners engaging in interactions and interventions which focus on the needs of the person within their context. Caring also includes making use of an evidence-based approach to providing the right care, in a timely way, at every stage of life.

Collaboration with colleagues is an essential aspect of providing high-quality care, as each professional brings unique skills and tools to the team. See also the **multidisciplinary team**.

Communication is 'central to successful caring relationships and to effective team working. Listening is as important as what we say and do' (Department of Health, 2012, p. 13).

Competence involves using skills, knowledge, and expertise in carrying out accurate assessments and delivering effective interventions relevant to the individual patient and based on research evidence.

Confidence in healthcare practice should never be misplaced. The NMC code (2018) states nursing care should be patient-centred and provides guidance on 'caring with confidence.'

Curiosity involves going beyond what is immediately obvious by observing, listening, asking questions, and reflecting on the information gathered.

Honesty is an essential quality in any person working in healthcare, due to the vulnerability of service users, many of whom will be living with long-term illnesses or conditions, which may make them fully or partially dependent on the care and support of others.

Non-discriminatory practice is a key value within a rights-based approach to care provision (British Institute for Human Rights, 2013), with the ideal being for all discrimination and inequality in healthcare provision to be prohibited, prevented, and eliminated.

Objectivity is central to being able to provide unbiased healthcare services, and practitioners should take great care not to use emotionally charged language in describing the responses and actions of others.

Privacy in healthcare is an important aspect of protecting dignity and maintaining respect, the erosion of which can lead to a sense of violation of the self.

Self-awareness of practitioners providing health and care services is integral to reflective practice, delivering person-centred care, and the therapeutic use of self to build relationships focused on a shared understanding of things which are important to the patient.

THEORIES

Ageism is a form of prejudice which influences how a person feels about other older people and getting old. Such prejudice can lead to thinking about older people in stereotypical ways or to acting in ways which are negative and discriminatory.

Avoiding assumptions: Stenhouse (2021, p. 27) states that practitioners 'must treat people as individuals, avoid making assumptions about them, recognise diversity and individual choice, and respect and uphold their dignity and human rights.'

Capacity in dementia, as in other people, is not a once-and-for-all assessment but is time and situation specific. Dementia does not itself exclude individuals from being able to make decisions for themselves.

Cognitive impairment refers to difficulties in thinking, learning, memory, judgement, and making decisions. Signs of cognitive impairment include memory loss and trouble concentrating, successful completion of tasks, understanding, remembering, following instructions, and solving problems.

Diagnostic overshadowing takes place when new symptoms are misattributed to an already diagnosed condition and leads to compromised patient care, including the risk of increased mortality.

Domains of dementia refer to the aspects of a person's life affected by dementia. The symptoms of dementia can be considered to have an impact on every aspect of a person's experience, including the physical, cognitive, intellectual, psychological, emotional, behavioural, sensory, functional, social, and spiritual domains of life and experience.

Family carers can experience a range of challenges and rewards in supporting a person living with dementia. Caring for a person living with dementia can cause family members to experience negative psychological and physical health outcomes (Alzheimer's Research UK, 2019).

Illness trajectories vary in different conditions. Dementia can lead to a long and variable disease process with progression for up to 6–8 years, involving the eventual impairment of all the domains of the person.

Labelling in dementia can depersonalise people and can have a significant impact on the way they feel about themselves as well as the way others behave towards them and decisions made about them.

Long-term management of symptoms, either of cancer itself or of the side effects or after-effects of an intervention, helps ensure that people regain and maintain quality of life following a cancer diagnosis. Self-management in the long term is particularly promoted in the NHS Long Term Plan (2019).

Memory in dementia is impacted in unique patterns according to the type and stage of dementia a person is living with and, therefore, what areas of the brain are impacted most by the death of brain cells. No two people, regardless of similarities in the type of dementia diagnosed or the areas of the brain affected, will experience memory changes in the same way.

Non-verbal communication includes gestures, facial expressions, movements, muscle tension, and posture, alongside the volume, tone, and pitch of vocalisations. Each person has an individual profile of non-verbal communication, although there may be some culturally and socially derived gestures and expressions which people from similar backgrounds share.

Occupational meaning relates to how occupations are seen in the culture in which a person belongs and allows others to create and associate the identity of a person through a particular set of occupations.

Patient perspectives on situations, and the understanding of health and care practitioners about these, are central to being able to provide person-centred assessments and interventions.

Perspectives on reality relate to an approach to understanding everyday reality in which each person is seen as having a unique perspective, thus recognising that objective truth for events has limits and that no one individual can claim to see or recall the situation precisely as it is experienced by others.

Practitioner resilience of individuals is formed as part of the wider resilience of teams, organisations, and the wider community to respond to and recover from difficult circumstances. Resilience should not be put down exclusively to the capacity of individuals to respond to stress.

Quality of life in dementia is difficult to define, due to it being subjective. Each person living with dementia is likely to have different ideas about what is needed for a good quality of life. The World Health Organisation defines quality of life as a person's perception of their well-being in relation to the fulfilment of personal goals and expectations (World Health Organisation, 2012).

Rank dynamics is a way of describing interactions and relationships between people at different levels within a hierarchical system, such as those often seen in healthcare systems.

Social stigma of dementia refers to dementia being seen as a social disgrace as outlined by Erving Goffman (1963). Goffman considered that stigma is an attribute that extensively discredits an individual, reducing him or her from someone seen as a whole person to someone seen as being tainted, who is discounted for the label that makes them stand out from others.

Stereotyping is the use of overgeneralised beliefs about groups of people, often based on assumptions made about specific characteristics thought to be held in common by all individuals in the group.

Unconscious bias is a form of social stereotyping about certain groups of people, formed outside of conscious awareness. Due to the tendency of humans to organise the social world by categorising people into groups, everyone holds unconscious beliefs about the various social and identity groups they come across.

APPROACHES

Activities of daily living (ADL) include all daily tasks and activities which contribute towards the well-being of the person. These activities can relate directly to personal care and maintaining health, domestic chores, exercise, and having periods of rest and leisure, as well as to activities which contribute indirectly to the fulfilment of wider goals – such as going shopping, using a computer, and texting or phoning friends.

Advocacy is a process through which it is ensured that every service user is heard and understood. It is an important concept in health and social care practice, sometimes being used as a way of describing the practitioner-patient relationship.

Assessment by observation can be carried out with or without validated tools, some of which consist of a straightforward checklist of, for example, actions, behaviours, activities, and environmental features to look out for. Checklists for observation tend to be either strengths-based or deficit-based.

Biomedicine focuses on identifying a specific cause for every illness and is biologically reductionist in the understanding offered of human health and disease. This contrasts with social and holistic approaches to health, which look beyond the malfunctioning body to gain an understanding of the whole person within their context.

Clinical supervision supports the provision of better-quality care for patients. This is achieved through discussions which support practice development and help practitioners to reflect on their decision-making and actions taken as well as potential strategies for future practice.

Communication with colleagues Is a key focus of professional development for practitioners at all stages of their careers.

Empathy is essential for providing person-centred care. It enables the person providing support to better understand the world from the perspective of the patient, and therefore to respond to their experience of service delivery with an individualised approach.

Explanation is a key facet of positive and compassionate healthcare practice, which supports patients to understand the purpose of appointments and what to expect from healthcare practitioners of different professions.

'Hello, my name is…' campaign: Dr Kate Granger, a medical doctor living with terminal illness, began the 'Hello, my name is' campaign with her husband in 2013 to encourage and remind healthcare staff about the importance of introductions in healthcare. Further information is available on the campaign website: https://www.hellomynameis.org.uk/.

Information finding is key to appropriate care planning in dementia care as well as in the provision of cancer services. Sources of information can variously include family and friends, experienced colleagues and research from peer-reviewed journals.

Multidisciplinary team working involves more than working alongside health practitioners from other professions or at a different stage of their careers. It also provides opportunities for taking into consideration different professional perspectives of relevance to decision-making, positive risk-taking, and reflection on and in practice, to improve patient outcomes.

Non-confrontational communication: Avoiding conflict as a communication strategy may delay facing a difficult situation. While beneficial in removing heated arguments from the public eye and as a way of resolving disputes professionally, there may be a risk of avoiding opportunities to resolve the conflict in the long term.

Occupational assessment involves identifying a person's strengths and barriers in areas of life which are important to them, as well as the spaces that surround them and how they occupy their time. In acute healthcare, this often involves assessing aspects of self-care and other activities of daily living.

Person-centred practice is an approach to working with people which provides dignity, respect, and choice. 'This denotes a shift away from routinised and task-oriented care practices in formal organisational settings' (Scales et al., 2017, p. 237).

Professional decision-making requires a non-judgemental approach to avoid making premature judgements or assumptions, which could impact on their decisions and so affect future actions and care planning in detrimental ways (Nibbelink and Brewer, 2018).

Professionalism leads to 'the consistent provision of safe, effective, person-centred outcomes that support people and their families and carers to achieve an optimal status of health and well-being' (NMC, 2016, p. 3).

Questioning in communication, when approached with an open mind and using open questions, can help to avoid conflict and to resolve differences in opinion professionally.

Reflective practice: The NMC and HCPC require reflection as part of the process of maintaining up-to-date and safe practice. A range of reflective models can be used to support the process of reflection.

Reflection on action is an effective starting point for improving professional practice in health and social care.

Shared decision-making focuses on including patients in all decisions about their own lives so that their voices are heard and their individual preferences understood and fully represented in any decision-making process which takes place.

Strengths-based practice enables family members and the person living with dementia to move beyond what can be experienced as an overwhelming sense of devastation following a diagnosis of dementia to focus on their individual and group resilience, alongside the enduring skills and attributes of the person diagnosed with dementia.

Supported decision-making often takes place in collaboration with family, friends, and professionals and involves providing support where there are gaps in understanding or ability, rather than overtaking an individual's autonomy or disempowering them by making decisions for them.

Teamwork plays an essential role in providing holistic care, as health-care assistants, support workers, doctors, nurses, occupational therapists, social workers, psychologists, and clinical support workers collaborate to provide quality joined-up holistic care.

The person in context, as seen at any moment in their patient journey, can paint a unique picture of their skills, abilities, and difficulties. Some environments are socially, physically and sensorially more difficult to navigate than others, and this needs to be taken into consideration when carrying out assessments.

Valuing experience from across a person's lifespan rather than just seeing the person as they are in the here and now helps in recognising the importance in the present of things which have happened in the past and helps to contribute to maintaining self-respect and a sense of dignity as the person shares an often-rich life history which may include many achievements.

Whole person care involves responding to the needs and strengths of the whole person, including influences on their physical, social, psychological, and spiritual well-being, both now and in the past, while embedding the principles of person-centred care into every intervention.

Working with care partners helps to provide a clearer picture of the strengths and struggles a patient may be experiencing. Being mindful of carer stress can help prevent the unsuccessful or damaging discharge of patients.

MODELS

Family of dementias: The term 'dementia' refers to a wide-ranging group of brain diseases, all of which lead to progressive cognitive impairment. The type (or types) of dementia affecting any individual is determined by where in the brain the disease process begins but more particularly by the mechanism of disease which is destroying brain cells. The most common type of dementia is Alzheimer's dementia, with Vascular dementia, dementia with Lewy bodies, and front-temporal dementia being other common types. Over 200 types of neurological impairment have been identified as belonging under the umbrella of the family of dementias.

Stages of dementia are often identified as early, middle, and late, or sometimes as being recognised across seven stages, up to the point of death. It is worth noting that no individual is likely to demonstrate all signs of cognitive deterioration according to a delineated progression through stages, as each person living with dementia is unique in terms of how dementia affects them and how well they can adapt to progressive cognitive impairment.

Symptoms of dementia are closely associated with symptoms of **cognitive impairment**. However, a person-centred understanding of social interactions, personality, the person's present health, their life history, and their interpretation of the neurological and cognitive changes they are experiencing all contribute to how each individual experiences the symptoms of dementia. For this reason, no two people will experience dementia in the same way.

Types of memory: Memory can be understood in terms of models which enable the conceptualisation of how it works. For example, it can be seen from diverse angles as having types, stages, and processes. The two types of memory (explicit memory and implicit memory) and the three major memory stages (sensory, short-term, and long-term) were originally outlined by Atkinson and Shiffrin (1968).

Validated assessments using standardised tools are essential for carrying out objective assessments. However, much of the time, even standardised tools can be influenced by subjective factors in assessment, such as the beliefs of the person being assessed about the purposes of the assessment, which will influence the answers they provide, as well as the practitioner's understanding of the need to use assessment tools in the way they were designed to be used.

References

Alzheimer's Research UK (2019) *Dementia in the Family: The Impact on Carers*. Available at: https://www. alzheimersresearchuk.org/wp-content/uploads/2019/09/Dementia-in-the-Family-The-impact-on-carers1.pdf (Accessed 27th May 2024).

Alzheimer's Society (2024) Available at: https://www.alzheimers.org.uk/get-support/legal-financial/making-decisions-mental-capacity-dementia (Accessed 27th May 2024).

Atkinson, R.C. and Shiffrin, R.M. (1968) Human Memory: A Proposed System and Its Control Processes. In K Spence (Ed.) *The Psychology of Learning and Motivation* (Vol 2). Oxford: Academic Press.

British Institute of Human Rights (2013) *The Difference It Makes: Putting Human Rights at the Heart of Health and Social Care*. London: BIHR. Available at: putting_human_rights_at_heart_of_health_and_care.pdf (bihr.org.uk) (Accessed 27th May 2024).

Dementia UK (2022) Available at: https://www.dementiauk.org/information-and-support/financial-and-legal-support/mental-capacity-and-decision-making/ (Accessed 27th May 2024).

Department of Health (2012) *Compassion in Practice; Nursing, Midwifery and Care Staff; Our Vision and Strategy*, London: Gateway reference 18479.

Farhana, N., Peckham, A., Marani, H., Roerig, M. and Marchildon G. (2023) The Social Construction of Dementia: Implications for Healthcare Experiences of Caregivers and People Living with Dementia. *Journal of Patient Experience*, 2023;10. Available at: https://doi.org/10.1177/23743735231211066.

Farre, A. and Rapley, T. (2017) The New Old (and Old New) Medical Model: Four Decades Navigating the Biomedical and Psychosocial Understandings of Health and Illness. *Healthcare*, 5(4):88. Available at: https://doi.org/10.3390/healthcare5040088.

Goffman, E. (1963/*1990) Stigma: Notes on the Management of Spoiled Identity*, London: Penguin.

Kydd, A. and Fleming, A. (2015) Ageism and Age Discrimination in Health Care: Fact or Fiction? A Narrative Review of the Literature. *Maturitas*, 81(4): 432–438.

McCormack, B., Bulley, C., McCance, T., McMillan, A., Martin, S. and Brown, D. (2021) *Fundamentals of Person-Centred Healthcare Practice*, Oxford: Wiley-Blackwell.

NHS (2019) *The NHS Long Term Plan*. Available at: https://www.longtermplan.nhs.uk/ (Accessed 28th May 2024).

Nibbelink, C.W. and Brewer, B.B. (2018) Decision-Making in Nursing Practice: An Integrative Literature Review. *Journal of Clinical Nursing*, 27(5–6): 917–928.

NMC (2016) Enabling Professionalism in Nursing and Midwifery Practice, Available at: https://www.nmc.org.uk/globalassets/sitedocuments/other-publications/enabling-professionalism.pdf (Accessed 28th May 2024).

NMC (2018) *The Code*. Available online at The Code: Professional standards of practice and behaviour for nurses, midwives and nursing associates – The Nursing and Midwifery Council (nmc.org.uk) (Accessed 28th May 2024).

Scales, K., Bailey, S., Middleton, J. and Schneider, J. (2017) Power, Empowerment, and Person-Centred Care: Using Ethnography to Examine the Everyday Practice of Unregistered Dementia Care Staff. *Sociology of Health & Illness*, 39: 227–243.

Stenhouse, R. (2021) Understanding equality and diversity in nursing practice. *Nursing Standard* (Royal College of Nursing, Great Britain), 36(2): 27–33. Available at: https://doi.org/10.7748/ns.2020.e11562.

Swift, H.J., Drury, L. and Lamont, R.A. (2016) The Perception of Ageing and Age Discrimination. *Other*. British Medical Association.

World Health Organisation (2012) *The World Health Organization Quality of Life (WHOQOL)*. Available at: https://www.who.int/toolkits/whoqol (Accessed 27th May 2024).

Case study 2
Sandra: mother knows best … or does she?

Rebekah Hill

Background

I first met Sandra in the gastroenterology outpatient department about a month ago. She had been referred by her general practitioner (GP) for further investigations following
a history of feeling unwell and developing jaundice. At
52 years old, Sandra is divorced and the sole carer for her
three children, aged 23, 20, and 17 years old. The children
still live at home, with the oldest two working locally and
the younger child being at college. Sandra's divorce has
been traumatic for her and serves as an unwanted end to a
26-year marriage. Sandra has been low in mood since the
divorce and attributed many of her initial clinical symptoms
to a low mood following the relationship split.

As the registered nurse covering the outpatients' clinic, I
sit in on Sandra's first appointment while the consultant
explains the investigation process and the possible diagnostic outcomes, one of which is cholangiocarcinoma. I
am not convinced that Sandra understands these potential
diagnostic outcomes. She looks glazed and is dismissive
when we ask if she has any questions. Not wanting to talk
about the situation, she quickly leaves the room at the end
of the consultation. I consider the potential shock of the
situation and am mindful of how individuals respond differently to bad news. I am also conscious that as a definitive
diagnosis has not yet been reached, no more can be done
at this stage.

> APPROACH: advanced communication

> THEORY: breaking bad news

> THEORY: grief

> MODEL: cancer care pathway

The worst outcome in this scenario would be cholangiocarcinoma (CCA), a rare type of cancer, also known as
bile duct cancer. It may not cause symptoms in the early
stages, but this depends on where the cancer is in the bile
ducts (either extrahepatic or intrahepatic). Sandra has mild
abdominal pain, feelings of depression and nausea but has
also noticed yellowing of her skin and the whites of her

DOI: 10.4324/9781003651758-2

eyes, which eventually triggered her visit to her GP. Having felt sad and lonely following her divorce, Sandra has developed a habit of having a glass of wine in the evening while watching television. Her initial thoughts, knowing that she is drinking well above the recommended maximum of 14 units a week (NHS, 2024), are that she has developed liver cirrhosis. Sandra's GP arranged an abdominal ultrasound, which showed a dilated bile duct. Her blood tests for liver function are also abnormal, triggering a request for a computerised tomography (CT) scan and then a magnetic resonance cholangiopancreatography (MRCP), which confirm the diagnosis of cholangiocarcinoma (Rushbrook et al., 2024). Sandra has no family history of cancer. Her parents are still alive and in good health.

Sandra's second consultation

A multidisciplinary team meeting has reviewed Sandra's investigations, and the diagnosis of stage 4 cholangiocarcinoma has been made. Since, at the point of presentation, metastatic disease is evident, the palliative care team is being involved.

At her second outpatient appointment, I am present again with the consultant. Sandra comes into the clinic room alone; she sits down opposite the gastroenterology consultant and looks up at him with a sad expression and tears in her eyes. 'So, it looks like my number's up,' she says, wringing her hands together tightly in her lap.

'What makes you say that, Sandra?'.

'Well, you asked me to bring someone with me today and that can never be a good thing, can it?' Sandra's manner of speech seems abrupt as she leans towards the consultant and looks directly at him. 'Plus, you have the world and his wife in the room – come to see the glowing woman.' Sandra comes across as almost hostile at this point.

I become aware that the room is somewhat crowded with the consultant, me, and a medical student present. I feel annoyed at myself for not explaining this to Sandra before she entered. We usually check whether the patient minds a medical student being present, but only once the patient is in the room, which would make it difficult for some people to say they would rather they were not there. I have left it for the consultant to check whether patients are comfortable with this at the start of appointments and feel guilty for not considering this. I make a mental note to talk to the consultant about this and, at the very least, to put a poster up in the clinic to explain that a medical student may be present with a request to tell the nurse if they do not wish to be seen with a student present.

VALUE: privacy

VALUE: consent

APPROACH: team working

THEORY: ethical decision-making

Another issue troubling me is Sandra's expression of herself as 'the glowing woman.' I assume she is referring to her jaundice but plan to check this before the appointment ends.

VALUE: clear communication

The consultant puts Sandra's notes on one side of the desk and leans forward to speak with her. As I regularly work with this consultant, I am familiar with his use of the SOLER technique (sit squarely, lean towards the other, eye contact, relax). This is a way to break bad news that takes the patient back to the beginning of the story and walks them through chronologically, from there to the present day. It is a gentle approach that enables the practitioner to take the patient with them through the presenting symptoms, any worries at the time, the investigations, and results. I am equally aware that other models for breaking bad news and for advanced communication exist.

APPROACH: advanced communication

APPROACH: effective listening

THEORY: breaking bad news

APPROACH: empathy

MODEL: Sage and Thyme

'You may remember when we met a few weeks ago Sandra, that we were worried about some of your initial test results and wanted to find out more.' The consultant speaks with a hushed voice and looks directly at Sandra, his head slightly to one side.

THEORY: breaking bad news

'Well, we have done several more investigations Sandra and have confirmed that you have cancer in your bile duct. It is an unusual cancer, and we know this will be a shock to you.' He continues, 'I know we mentioned that we

VALUE: sensitivity

were worried when we last met that the cancer might have advanced. Some of the test results show that our fears have been confirmed. I'm afraid, there is already spread of the cancer Sandra.'

Sandra shrugs her shoulders, 'Oh well, I sort of knew you were going to tell me the worst.'

'Sandra, I notice you have come to clinic on your own,' says the consultant. 'Is there anyone we can contact to be with you?'

VALUE: support

'No thanks. There's just me and the kids now, since he left us.'

APPROACH: holistic patient care and support

'Can we help you with the children Sandra, would you like us to talk to them with you?' asks the consultant.

'Absolutely not,' Sandra quickly replies. 'They aren't to know; they have been through enough. There is no way I am telling them or letting you either.' Sandra is firm in her reply and has an angry expression on her face.

THEORY: grief

'They all think I hit the sherry – let them think that. I heard someone talking about me in the Tesco queue the other day – looking in my shopping trolley at the wine and making comments about me having had enough of that! I hear them. It's because of the yellow. It's worse in some lights. I make sure I keep the lamps on at home and keep the main light off as much as I can. The kids see me every day, so I don't think they notice as much. Let them think that I've hit the bottle. That's better than knowing this.' Sandra seems sad now, with an unusual softness in her voice that resonates with defeat. She leans back in her chair and looks at the ground.

THEORY: stigma and discrimination

'What do you think the children might say Sandra, if you did tell them?' The consultant gently asks.

APPROACH: information finding

'Well, we won't know – because I'm not going to tell them. Not yet anyway,' Sandra replies abruptly. She continues: 'People think I'm rubbish; they think I'm a boozer because of the yellow – you should see the looks I get. I only go out when I must now. I can't stand the looks and the whispers, the talking.'

'I wonder how that makes you feel Sandra,' asks the consultant.

APPROACH: open communication

'It makes me feel rubbish. Just rubbish,' replies Sandra. 'It's bad enough that I have this situation – never mind everybody knowing about it. Well, they think they know about it. As though I deserve it because they think I am a drinker. Well, I can tell you – no one deserves this. No one. I feel sorry for people with drink problems – they drink for a reason – and they don't deserve to be treated like they are lepers or something.'

THEORY: labelling

'Is that what you think Sandra – that the jaundice makes people treat you differently?'

VALUE: respect and non-judgemental care

'It's not what I think – it's what I know,' Sandra replies. 'That's the worst of it – feeling labelled and judged. People think you are a bad person; they assume you are a drinker.'

The consultant responds to Sandra: 'I must tell you – it is common for people with jaundice to feel like this.' He pauses, and she looks up at him. 'It's really common. Many of my patients tell me the same thing, and it's a very well recognised situation within the medical literature that people with jaundice are treated with discrimination. Jaundice is a stigmatised symptom, Sandra; it relates to people having unfair beliefs about the cause of jaundice, and people are treated differently as a response to these mistakenly held beliefs. That's discrimination – and to experience it must feel awful.'

THEORY: stigma and discrimination

APPROACH: empathy

VALUE: compassion

'So, others have said that too? Other patients who see you have had the same?' Sandra asks.

'Yes Sandra, sadly it's a thing I hear a lot.'

APPROACH: sharing experiences

Sandra looks thoughtful and seems to be comforted by what the consultant has said. A long pause follows.

Focus on the children

'May we go back to the children Sandra?' asks the consultant. 'Why do you feel they are better not to know about your diagnosis?'

I am thinking that Sandra may be robbing herself of an important source of support from her children. Not telling them prevents them from supporting her as well as preventing them from coming to terms with the ultimate loss of their mum. The children might have regrets, things they could have said or done differently if only they knew. Not knowing might also delay the bereavement process.

I am concerned for Sandra, who is trying to cope with this situation all alone; it must be unbearable for her. I know they say 'mother knows best', but I am unsure that, in this situation, she does. Yet I also know that I need to support Sandra in her decision-making, or at least not to contradict or judge it. I need to advocate for Sandra, who knows her children and home situation better than anyone else.

I feel compelled to speak out. 'You are coping with a lot on your own Sandra'. The consultant and Sandra both look around at me – I have been silent up until this point in the appointment. I blush slightly at the sudden attention.

'Would you consider letting us try to help Sandra? Would you consider letting us refer you to the Family Support Centre? They work from the Palliative Care Centre'. I am worried that using the words 'palliative care' might make Sandra feel uncomfortable – as it has connotations of hopelessness. I am mindful that perhaps I am judging this situation from my own perspective, from my own values, rather than from Sandra's, but I firmly believe that Sandra should not have to cope alone with this situation. I hope she will accept help from the counselling service, which can help her break the news to her children.

After a long silence, Sandra looks up at me and nods. 'Ok then, I will think about the Family Support Team, if you think it will help.'

'Yes Sandra, I think it will help,' I reply, feeling relieved that Sandra is willing to consider sources of support for herself and her children.

Reflection

This scenario leaves me feeling uncomfortable for several reasons. Could I have done more to support her experiences of stigma and discrimination? People with cholangiocarcinoma are known to have low health-related quality of life scores as well as anxiety, depression, and self-isolation (Rushbrook et al., 2024). Jaundice-causing experiences of stigma are well documented in research (Marta et al., 2022). I felt disappointed with myself for not tackling this issue with Sandra at her first appointment by asking her how she felt about her jaundice or if she had experienced any discrimination or stigma. Although we had hoped, of course, that the jaundice was caused by a gallstone, which might easily be removed and so resolve the situation.

People presenting with cholangiocarcinoma typically present too late for surgical resection or transplant, which are currently the only curative options (Rushbrook et al., 2024). Over 95% of cholangiocarcinoma cases are diagnosed in people over 50 years old, with an average age at diagnosis of 75 years (Rushbrook et al., 2024).

I am conscious of the need to offer support to Sandra but am also aware that until a definitive diagnosis is available, it is difficult to know what support will be best. Although cancer support services exist, they tend to focus on a specific type, site, or location, so until a diagnosis was established, support was lacking. The Alan Morement Memorial Fund (AMMF) is the UK's only cholangiocarcinoma charity that offers much in the way of support, and this would be available to Sandra following confirmation of her diagnosis.

Whether the approach the consultant used was the most effective way to communicate is also worth reflecting on. It is always pertinent to reflect on whether enough space has been left for asking questions, whether we have listened well enough to our patients and whether we have allowed them to explore and disclose concerns fully and without interruption.

Difficulties associated with telling a person a cancer diagnosis are much discussed in research and theory, but considering this from a patient's perspective is essential. Although many patients prefer to be told their diagnosis by a physician in the presence of a family member (Arbabi et al., 2014), this is not always the case. Some evidence suggests that disclosing more detailed information about cancer for terminally ill people can contribute to improving the quality of communication (Nakajima et al., 2015).

Equally, there are no hard and fast right or wrong ways of telling children about a parent's cancer diagnosis. This is an understudied area within healthcare research (Muñoz Sastre et al., 2016). I remind myself not to judge based on my own values and opinions. I am aware of the need to do several things going forward: to respect Sandra's decisions and autonomy, not to make assumptions about her children's ability to cope, and to appreciate and empower her around her experiences of stigma and discrimination due to her jaundice.

Questions for reflection and discussion

Explore the key issues raised in the above scenario as you answer the following six questions:

1. Describe how a healthcare practitioner can support people with having difficult conversations.

2. Identify models of communication that can help support breaking bad news and explain their effectiveness.

3. Describe the stages of bereavement seen in Sandra's situation and in those of patients and their families with whom you have worked.

4. How would you approach this situation in ways which might improve communication with Sandra?

5. Reflect on the causes of stigma and discrimination, discussing how they might impact individuals and their families in the shorter and longer terms.

6. Identify and explain the rationale for ways health practitioners and healthcare teams can support and empower people experiencing stigma or discrimination.

Further reading

Cancer Research UK. *Talking to Children about Cancer*. https://www.cancerresearchuk.org/about-cancer/coping/mental-health-cancer/talking-children

Goffman, E. (1963) *Stigma. Notes on the Management of Spoiled Identity*. London, Penguin.

Mannix, K. (2019) *With the End in Mind: How to Live and Die Well*. London, Harper Collins.

Mannix, K. (2021) *Listen. How to Find the Words for Tender Conversations*. London, Harper Collins.

Tyrrell, P., Harberger, S., Schoo, C. and Siddiqui, W. (2023) *Kübler-Ross Stages of Dying and Subsequent Models of Grief*. https://www.ncbi.nlm.nih.gov/books/NBK507885/

Further information

VALUES

Advocacy means getting support from another person to help you express your views and wishes and to help you stand up for your rights. It can be common for healthcare practitioners to advocate for a person by representing or supporting their perspective and interests.

Clear communication is one of the core NHS values, to ensure that communication is clear, concise, concrete, correct, coherent, complete, and courteous.

Compassion is a value manifest in seeing and understanding the suffering of others. It is one of the core values of the NHS. Compassion relates to understanding how care is given through developing relationships based on empathy, respect, and dignity. It is described as 'intelligent kindness' and is essential to understanding how people perceive their care.

Consent is essential for ethical and legal medical treatment, but importantly the consent must be informed – patients must understand and agree to testing and treatment before it can proceed. The consent must be clear, continuous, coercion-free, and conscious.

Non-judgemental care acknowledges individuality and holism and all aspects of people's lives. The values involved in non-judgemental care are acceptance, empathy, and sincerity. Acceptance is about respecting the person's feelings, experiences, and values, even though they may differ from yours. The Nursing and Midwifery Council (2018) stresses that nurses must practise in a holistic, non-judgemental, caring, and sensitive manner that avoids assumptions and supports social inclusion, recognises and respects individual choice, and acknowledges diversity.

Privacy is respecting the right to be left alone, free from intrusion or interference. In healthcare, we think about information privacy as the right to have control over how your personal information is used or collected. Privacy is about respecting individuals and their right to keep something private by choosing to limit disclosure of some information.

Respect is showing due regard for the feelings, wishes or rights of others. Treating people with respect demonstrates that you think they have worth. In healthcare, having respect for others is an essential value to be displayed, shown by politeness, honour, and care towards others.

Sensitivity is an important value to maintain in healthcare since being sensitive in communication is considering what is said and how it is said and being receptive to how the other person is engaging with you in the conversation, thus allowing you the opportunity to refine your message and its delivery.

Support involves taking part of a burden to assist or encourage a person to continue. Having psychological and emotional support is important when people are vulnerable.

THEORIES

Breaking bad news can be understood as any news that changes a person's view of the future in a negative way. A nurse cannot judge what constitutes bad news for an individual and must be aware that any news has the potential to alter an individual's view of themselves or their future. There are several accepted ways to break bad news. These methods include using common formats of structured listening to what the patient knows and wants to know, giving information in understandable amounts, reacting to the news, and checking for understanding.

Cancer risks can be categorised into internal or external factors. External factors may include chemicals, radiation, and viruses, while internal factors can include hormones, immune conditions, and inherited mutations.

Deflection is a defence mechanism characterised by redirecting a conversation away from a challenging topic or issue to something less emotionally tense. Deflection can manifest in numerous ways, such as changing the subject, asking a question, making a joke, or even becoming defensive or aggressive.

Ethical decision-making is a cognitive process where people consider ethical rules, principles, or guidelines when making decisions. There are four main principles of ethics: autonomy, beneficence, justice, and non-maleficence. Each patient has the right to make their own decisions based on their own beliefs and values.

Grief theory relates to the five stages of grief developed by the psychiatrist Kübler-Ross (2005). The theory suggests that we go through five distinct stages after the loss of a loved one. These stages are denial, anger, bargaining, depression, and finally acceptance.

Help seeking theory postulates that people follow a series of predictable steps to seek help when needed. It is a series of well-ordered and purposeful cognitive and behavioural steps, each leading to specific types of solutions.

Hopelessness is a feeling or state of despair. Hopelessness, by definition, is the belief that things are not going to get better or that you cannot succeed.

Judgement involves forming an opinion based on comparisons, insight, or understanding after thinking carefully about something. It is essential to be mindful of personal bias because a judgement is an opinion based on personal perception, and implicit bias can exist.

Labelling draws attention to the idea that the experience of having an illness has both social and physical consequences for an individual. Labelling, stereotyping, and prejudice involve treating people differently because of assumptions made about a person or group of people based on their differences.

Stigma and discrimination are distinct. Stigma is when someone perceives you in a negative way because of a particular characteristic or attribute (such as skin colour, cultural background, disability, or mental illness). When someone treats you in a negative way because of a characteristic, this is discrimination.

APPROACHES

Advanced communication is having the knowledge of effective communication beyond basic communication abilities. Advanced communication skills enable individuals to articulate ideas with clarity, purpose, and efficiency to maximise their impact on the person. It enables an individual to engage in complex social interactions with others across a range of topics, which helps to develop relationships.

Effective listening means not just understanding the words or the information being communicated but also understanding the emotions the speaker is trying to convey.

Empathy is an approach reflecting a willingness to understand and prioritise the social and emotional needs of another person during times of difficulty.

Family-centred care is a way of providing services which assure the health and well-being of children and their families through respectful partnerships of family members with professionals.

Holistic patient care and support involves treating the whole patient, not just the disease, and is fundamental to person-centred practice. Understanding the physical, emotional, and spiritual needs of patients can help providers provide optimal care and improve outcomes.

Information finding recognises that if an individual finds out about their illness and treatment, it can help to give them a feeling of control, which can in turn help them to feel more confident about the future.

Open communication is the ability to express your thoughts freely while interacting with other people. In healthcare, it refers to the ability of practitioners to share and receive feedback, provide ideas and suggestions, and raise concerns, which makes them active participants in the treatment process.

Person-centred care focuses care on the needs of the individual, ensuring that their preferences, needs, and values guide clinical decisions and that services are provided in a respectful way.

Sharing experiences enhances our feelings of belonging, connectedness, and a sense of meaning. Additionally, it can boost self-esteem and decrease feelings of depression, anxiety, and isolation.

Teamworking is vital for successful healthcare delivery. A successful team is one which recognises everyone's unique skills and strengths, helping each team member to contribute to achieve shared goals.

MODELS

Cancer care pathways are tools used by cancer care physicians to make the best cancer treatment recommendations for the type of cancer diagnosed. They incorporate evidence-based cancer treatment protocols that assure the individual will receive the same high standards of cancer care, no matter where they are treated in the UK.

Sage and Thyme (Connolly et al., 2010) is a model which consists of firstly using four steps of SAGE: Setting, Ask, Gather, and Emphasise – each with an emphasis on the importance of listening with a view to enabling patients to feel calmer and more settled. THYME is then used to empower the patient: Talked, you can ask who they have talked to about their concern. Help, did talking help? What do you think will help? ME: Is there anything I can do to help?

References

Arbabi, M., Rozdar, A., Taher, M., Shirzad, M., Arjmand, M., Ansari, S. and Mohammadi, M.R. (2014) Patients' Preference to Hear Cancer Diagnosis. *Iranian Journal of Psychiatry*, 9(1): 8–13.

Connolly, M., Perryman, J., McKenna, Y., Orford, J., Thomson, L., Shuttleworth, J. and Cocksedge, S. (2010) SAGE & THYME: A Model for Training Health and Social Care Professionals in Patient-focussed Support. *Patient Education Counselling*, 79(1): 87–93.

Kübler-Ross, E. and Kessler, D. (2005) On Grief and Grieving: Finding the Meaning of Grief through the Five Stages of Loss. Available at: https://grief.com/images/pdf/5%20Stages%20of%20Grief.pdf (Accessed 13th June 2024).

Marta, C., Perez-Guasch, M., Sola, E., Cervera, M., Martinez, S., Juanola, A., Ma, A., Avitabile, E., Napoleone, L., Pose, E., Graupera, I., Honrubia, M. and Korenjak, M. (2022) Stigmatization Is Common in Patients with Non-alcoholic Fatty Liver Disease and Correlates with Quality of Life. *PLOS ONE*. Available at: https://journals.plos.org/plosone/article?id=10.1371/journal.pone.0265153.

Muñoz Sastre, M.T., Sorum, P.C. and Mullet, E. (2016) Telling Children Their Mother Is Seriously Ill or Dying: Mapping French People's Views. *Child: Care, Health & Development*, 42(1): 60–67.

Nakajima, N., Kusumoto, K., Onishi, H. and Ishida, M. (2015) Does the Approach of Disclosing More Detailed Information of Cancer for the Terminally Ill Patients Improve the Quality of Communication Involving Patients, Families, and Medical Professionals? *American Journal of Hospice & Palliative Medicine*, 32(7): 776–782.

NHS (2024) Alcohol Units. Available at: https://www.nhs.uk/live-well/alcohol-advice/calculating-alcohol-units/#:~:text=men%20and%20women%20are%20advised,as%2014%20units%20a%20week (Accessed 13th June 2024).

Rushbrook, S., Kendall, T., Zen, Y., Albazaz, R., Manoharan, P., Pereira, S., Sturgess, R., Davidson, B., Malik, H., Manas, D., Heaton, N., Prasad, K., Bridgewater, J., Valle, J., Goody, R., Hawkins, M., Prentice, W., Morement, H., Walmsley, M. and Khan, S. (2024) British Society of Gastroenterology Guidelines for the Diagnosis and Management of Cholangiocarcinoma. *Gut*, 73, 16–46.

Case study 3
Ravi: a time to dialyse and a time to die

Rebekah Hill and Emma Watts

Ravi's clinical background

Ravi felt a breast lump when he was 64 years old. He had noticed a swelling in his armpit but thought nothing of it, assuming it was a cyst and being unaware that men could get breast cancer. Breast cancer in men is rare; only 370 men per year are diagnosed in the UK, compared to 55,500 women (Cancer Research UK, 2024).

Ravi's wife eventually persuaded him to go to the GP when he developed a nipple discharge, which he had dismissed as sweat. A mammogram and biopsy diagnosed Ravi's breast cancer but did not explain the nausea and tiredness that he had also been experiencing for some months. Ravi had magnetic resonance imaging (MRI) and positron emission tomography (PET) scans which confirmed his worst fears: the cancer had spread to his bones. Ravi has Stage 4 breast cancer with rib and pelvic metastases. He has received chemotherapy and radiotherapy to keep both in check under a pathway of palliative care (NICE, 2017).

Ravi also has chronic kidney disease (CKD), which is a long-term condition whereby the kidneys are unable to function as well as they should. The kidneys are life-sustaining organs responsible for performing essential functions such as regulating blood osmolarity and pH, regulating blood volume and blood pressure, producing hormones, metabolic conversion, and excreting metabolic waste (Rainey, 2023; Thomas, 2014). CKD involves the gradual loss of kidney function. This could be due to damage or abnormalities in the structure or function (or both) of the kidneys for more than 3 months (NICE, 2024). Individuals with CKD may not present with symptoms of kidney disease until the later stages of disease progression.

Those with CKD will not recover their kidney function. Once diagnosed, an individual is categorised into a stage of

DOI: 10.4324/9781003651758-3

disease progression. CKD Stage 1 represents mild kidney damage, whilst CKD Stage 5 represents severe damage, also known as end-stage renal failure (ESRF). The rate of disease progression varies from person to person; some individuals will remain stable with mild kidney damage for years and will never reach ESRF. Others, whose kidney disease progresses more rapidly, will reach CKD Stage 5, as has happened to Ravi (Kidney Research UK, 2023).

Treatment for CKD depends on the severity of the disease. In the earlier stages of CKD, lifestyle changes and medication may slow the progression of the disease, yet in ESRF, treatment options include renal replacement therapy, a renal transplant, or conservative management.

Ravi's story

VALUE: respect

APPROACH: holistic patient care

THEORY: renal replacement therapy

As I enter the side room, I can see that Ravi is sleeping. I approach the side of the bed and place my hand on his hand to gently wake him, calling out his name. I can feel that his hand is cold, and the skin has become thin and withdrawn to reveal his veins and the skeletal shape of his hand. He looks so frail, and I want to let him sleep, but I also know this is the best time of day to dialyse him, when there's a medical team around to provide support should he become unwell during his treatment.

Ravi smiles and looks up at me, 'Is it time to hook me up?'

'If that's ok with you, I'll just set the dialysis machine up and then we can get started. The doctors don't want any fluid removal today, just dialysis as you're a little dehydrated.'

Ravi closes his eyes again, 'I'll just do three hours today; I want to be off the machine before Pippa comes to visit so she can take me outside for a cigarette.'

I smile as I say, 'Ravi, you know your treatment is four hours. You're not going to feel well if we continue to shorten your sessions, not to mention that you're on oxygen and you shouldn't be smoking.' I've known Ravi for 4 years; he was the first person I ever dialysed, and he's seen me grow from a newly qualified nurse through to motherhood and marriage – I feel I have earned his respect and am able to talk to him candidly.

APPROACH: *professional relationships*

Ravi does not respond; he has fallen asleep again. As I move around the bed, he opens his eyes and reaches out for my hand, holding it tightly. I think this is a bit strange because usually he would reply with a witty response. I can hear my heart beating, and I am bothered that he holds my hand so tightly. The tone of the room has completely changed, and I feel a little sad because at that moment all I can see is a once proud and energetic man, now tired and weary.

MODEL: *effective communication*

Once the dialysis machine is ready, I prepare my trolley and start to clean the dialysis catheter. Ravi is staring out of the window, but his view is far from interesting; it is just a small brick courtyard.

Still looking out the window, Ravi says, 'How long do you think I could live without dialysis? I think I'm ready to stop all of this. I'm tired and I'm dying, I'm on borrowed time, the dialysis is just prolonging the end.'

And just like that we are having one of the biggest discussions a nurse can ever have with a patient.

'Do you think you could be feeling like this because you're unwell at the moment? You've got a nasty chest infection, you're tired and I'm sure it just feels overwhelming right now, being in hospital' I suggest. 'We're in and out of your room all day to either give you antibiotics, dialysis treatment or pain relief, we're not letting you rest much.'

VALUE: *honesty*

'How long have you known me? Four years? You know I'm not going to get better, and I need to be able to talk about my options.' Ravi was looking directly at me now.

I can feel tears welling up in my eyes but remain focused so that they do not overcome me.

'If you stop dialysis you will die. I can't tell you how long it would be because it's different for each person. Some people might die within a few days, others may die a week or so later. I really think that if you're considering dialysis withdrawal you should speak with Pippa and then the doctor. Please don't decide either way without having all the information you need to make the right decision.' I reply.

THEORY: advanced directives

Ravi's upper torso becomes slightly tense as he replies, 'I've tried talking to the doctors about it, but they always have a solution to how I'm feeling – more dialysis, more drugs. They tell me that stopping dialysis is further down the line and we should monitor how things go, but what they don't see is that I feel like I'm becoming less of a man and that's worse than lying in this bed waiting to die.'

I tell Ravi that if he wants to postpone his dialysis, perhaps until he's spoken with Pippa and the doctors, I can stop the treatment. He declines and agrees to the dialysis, and I wonder if it is because he knows he needs time to prepare his family and himself for the difficult discussions and decisions ahead.

VALUE: informed consent

MODEL: advocacy

I commence Ravi's treatment, make him comfortable in bed and promise to call the doctor and relay our conversation. When I'm able to leave, I go to the drugs room and cry, thinking about everything he has just told me. I feel a little broken by his words. I anticipate that the day will be full of difficult conversations, and I reflect upon the age-old dilemma that every renal nurse faces – a common question that we often ask ourselves, is there a time to die and a time to dialyse?

A colleague, and very trusted friend, walks into the drugs room.

'I've just answered Ravi's call bell, he looks grey – why are we still dialysing him. Poor man needs a holiday,' she says.

I wipe the tears away from under my eyes and chuckle. 'He wants to stop dialysis. I need to call the doctors and let them know. He seems quite accepting of the idea and he's battle-ready to stand his ground if they suggest a different treatment plan.'

My colleague relaxes into a pose that suggests we have time to discuss this further, and we do. We recall other patients who bravely made similar decisions, those who knew that dialysis was prolonging their death, not their quality of life.

APPROACH: peer support

I call the doctor, and he assures me he will review Ravi at lunchtime when Pippa comes to visit. I make sure that I loiter by the reception as the lunch trays are being handed out, and I feel annoyed at myself because I did not consider that talking about death and dying at lunchtime is probably quite inconsiderate.

THEORY: reflection

As the doctor comes onto the ward, he anticipates that I have been waiting for him. With hands in his pockets, he casually asks me, 'Is the wife here yet?'

He has irritated me already with this off-hand remark, so I reply sharply, 'Her name is Pippa.'

He looks embarrassed, and I am glad that he does, but he apologises, so I relent a little and give him a brief back-ground of how long Ravi has been on dialysis, his family circumstances and his current health concerns. The doctor reads through the medical notes before I interfere again and advise him that Ravi is a man who knows his own mind and will not be blinded by false possibilities. He asks if I want to join him for the discussion, but I decline. This private moment is for Ravi and his family, so I take a step back and respect their need for privacy and intimacy.

APPROACH: holistic patient care

VALUE: privacy

For two days, the medical team offers Ravi alternative antibiotic treatments and reduced dialysis therapy as an alternative to completely withdrawing from treatment. Ravi either refuses these offers or is found conveniently asleep when the doctors try to speak with him. He would be very much awake moments later, asking for a sneaky trip out-side for a cigarette.

Three days later Ravi dies, surrounded by his family and with his favourite music playing in the background.

MODEL: end-of-life care

With Ravi's death, I feel overwhelmed with feelings that I feel I should not have. I choke back tears when he is spoken of amongst the nursing team, because it is painful to acknowledge all the things he will never be part of, such as his granddaughter's wedding and a family holiday planned for a milestone birthday. What strikes me most is that I do not feel able to talk about my feelings because no one within the workplace recognises my grief. It has become accepted that I should just carry on with the job in front of me instead of processing an event that has impacted me emotionally and professionally. Does the fault lie with the system, or is it just an occupational hazard? We are so overwhelmed with bed flow that we put our own resilience to one side to provide patient care in the most demanding and challenging work circumstances.

VALUE: resilience

The week following his death, Ravi's family came to the ward to deliver thank you cards. Pippa hugs me tightly and thanks me for the years of being more than a dialysis nurse. As she pulls back, she whispers, 'He's at peace.' I sob. This was the permission I needed to cry.

THEORY: grief

Reflections

Renal nursing is a unique profession; the nurse-patient relationship is multifaceted, full of trust, empathy, compassion, resilience, and grief. It has both rewards and challenges. Dialysis patients often attend for treatment two to four times a week for sessions that last between three and four and a half hours. The act of physically preparing a patient for dialysis treatment is one of intimacy. From preparing the patient's dialysis access, close bodily contact is maintained between nurse and patient during the initial stages of treatment. A relationship of trust is fundamental, and patients must have faith in my ability to provide not only the technical aspects of life-sustaining treatment but also the emotional support and reassurance needed on this unpredictable treatment road.

I need to see the whole person and not just their diagnosis. Emotionally engaging with patients and recognising and understanding the psychological challenges of being dialysis dependent, I develop a better understanding of how to make them feel understood and supported, reducing their feelings of isolation and anxiety. Patients who feel truly listened to and understood are more likely to engage in their treatment plans and undertake greater responsibility in their own care.

Through the days, weeks, months, and years of dialysis treatment, I can come to feel responsible for patients' well-being. When patients become unwell and their disease progression worsens, I feel the burden of that. Whilst recognising the professional boundaries of a nurse-patient relationship, I also grieve for the person I knew and often sacrifice those emotions to better support the families left behind.

In the final days of Ravi's life, he simply slipped into sleep and then died. His death was so significant to my nursing career that I felt his absence for some time. Even now, I am reminded of the most trivial things. I might hear a patient arguing for help to go outside for a cigarette, and I remember how Ravi would disregard all safety guidelines when it came to smoking outside with his hand-held oxygen tank resting at his feet.

It is an emotive experience to be a renal nurse, and it's important to have opportunities to express and process grief. The psychological and emotional effects of patient loss amongst renal nurses are under-represented in research. I decided to take Ravi and me to a Schwartz round I had seen advertised in the hospital.

The death of Ravi was my first experience of a dialysis death. It has become a life-defining moment for me. Ravi's decision to withdraw from treatment poses an important question that we should consider amongst our patient population. Alongside patient education on the advantages and disadvantages of treatment, we should ask our patients to make their treatment wishes known through advanced directives when discussions around treatment efficacy need to be discussed. It seems that there is a time to dialyse and a time to die.

Questions for reflection and discussion

Explore the key issues raised in the above scenario as you answer the following six questions:

1. Explain what advanced directives are and when and why they might be useful.

2. Describe how healthcare practitioners can support patients and their families in dealing with advanced directives.

3. How do you think renal nurses can support each other in situations when patients die?

4. What stage of grief do you think Ravi had reached, and what led you to this decision?

5. Explain what a Schwartz round is, and how you think they can help renal nurses in these situations.

6. Think about how communication can be enhanced in ESRF and palliative care situations in relation to starting difficult conversations.

Further reading

Cousins, M., Bradshaw, J., and Bonner, A. (2020) Professional relationships between nephrology clinicians and patients: A systematic review. *Journal of Renal Care*, 46(4): 206–215.

Flanagan, E., Chadwick, R., Goodrich, J., Ford, C., and Wickens, R. (2019) Reflection for all healthcare staff: A national evaluation of Schwartz Rounds. *Journal of Interprofessional Care*, 34(1): 140–142.

Mannix, K. (2019) *With the End in Mind: How to Live and Die Well*. London: Harper Collins.

Mannix, K. (2021) *Listen. How to Find the Words for Tender Conversations*. London: Harper Collins.

Salyanarayana, V., Narothama, A., and Chaddie, D. (2021) *Chronic Kidney Disease*. National Center for Biotechnology Information. https://www.ncbi.nlm.nih.gov/books/NBK568778/.

Further information

VALUES

Informed consent is a process whereby people need to be given all the information required to make a fully informed decision about a medical procedure or treatment.

Privacy is the right to be alone, free from interference or intrusion.

Professional honesty involves telling the truth to people and showing adherence to moral and ethical principles that require nurses to have professional integrity and trustworthiness.

Resilience refers to the idea that professionals can bounce back from challenging situations and setbacks in a positive way, often emerging stronger than before. Resilience is seen as an important professional value and quality to cultivate.

Respect is about how people act towards each other, valuing a person's perspective, qualities, and context.

THEORIES

Advanced directives enable individuals to think about what they would like to happen if they lose the capacity to make informed decisions about their care.

Grief theory relates to a collection of ideas about how people experience and respond to grief after a loss, some suggesting there are stages to how people respond to death.

Reflection theory is based on looking back on an experience to learn from it. Often using a systematic approach as a model, reflection facilitates a way to explore experiences to allow growth and learning.

Renal replacement therapy is a treatment that replaces the function of the kidneys when they are not working properly. The techniques used include haemodialysis, peritoneal dialysis, and renal transplantation.

APPROACHES

Holistic patient care is a comprehensive approach to healthcare that considers the whole person, not just the symptom or illness. It is based on a mutual understanding of the physical, social, psychological, emotional, and spiritual dimensions of a person.

Peer support is an effective way of supporting colleagues who share similar experiences.

Professional relationships are connections between people in a professional setting; they are built on mutual trust and respect yet recognise that professional boundaries are present.

MODELS

Advocacy is an important aspect of being an effective health carer. Advocacy involves acting for others and helping them to have their voices and opinions heard when decisions are being made that affect them.

Effective communication is an essential skill of professional healthcare staff which involves conveying clear messages, actively listening to others, and providing constructive feedback. Effective communication involves verbal and non-verbal features.

End-of-life care is supporting people to have a good death, to be as pain and symptom-free as possible and to receive emotional and spiritual support which focuses on what matters to the individual.

References

Cancer Research UK (2024) *Breast Cancer in Men*. https://www.cancerresearchuk.org/about-cancer/breast-cancer/types/male-breast-cancer (Accessed 13th June 2024).

Kidney Research UK (2023) *Kidney Disease: A UK Public Health Emergency*. Economics-of-Kidney-Disease-full-report_accessible.pdf (kidneyresearchuk.org) (Accessed: 7th May 2024).

NICE (2017) *Breast Cancer Guidance. Advanced Breast Cancer: Diagnosis and Treatment.* https://www.nice.org.uk/hub/indevelopment/gid-hub10003 (Accessed 13th June 2024).

NICE (2024) *Chronic Kidney Disease: Assessment and Management* (NG203). https://www.nice.org.uk/guidance/ng203.

Rainey, H. (2023) Chronic kidney disease: Understanding its association with other long-term conditions. *Nursing Standard*, 3(23):1–5. doi: 10.7748/ns. 2023.e12081.

Thomas, N. (2014) *Renal Nursing: Care and Management of People with Kidney Disease.* 4th edn. Sussex: Wiley, Blackwell.

Case study 4
Claire: am I going to die?

Helen Humphrey and Marie O'Donovan

Claire's admission to the adolescent unit

Following her bone marrow transplant (BMT), 14-year-old Claire was transferred from the specialist regional BMT unit to a general unit for adolescents aged 12–18, where I work as a children's and young people's nurse. She is 110 days post-transplant, and the decision has been made to transfer Claire closer to home for further management and potential end-of-life care. Claire's mother Gill is a resident with her on the unit, and her father Josef visits daily. On handover from the regional centre, I was informed that her post-transplant period has been complicated by ongoing graft-versus-host disease (GVHD) and multiple serious infections. Despite aggressive treatment, Claire's condition has continued to deteriorate, showing signs of organ failure and a significant decline in her clinical status.

I understand that although the family are happy to be transferred closer to home, they are deeply distressed and refuse to accept the possibility of ceasing antimicrobial treatment. The handover from the BMT team suggests that this treatment has had limited effectiveness and the ongoing decline in her health will continue. The family have so far resisted discussions about parallel planning, which includes preparing for possible end-of-life care, and insist that Claire continues to be for full resuscitation with the option for admission to paediatric intensive care if needed. This is against the advice of the intensive care consultants.

Day 1 of admission – Anita's shift

Following the handover, I am allocated as the nurse caring for Claire and her family. This is my first meeting with them on the adolescent unit.

DOI: 10.4324/9781003651758-4

'Good morning, my name is Anita, I'm a staff nurse on the unit and will be your allocated nurse for the day shift today,' I say as an introduction.

I am surprised at Claire's mum's response, lacking the usual first meeting pleasantries, as she says, 'Can I ask how long you have worked here Anita, as I'm conscious that my daughter requires experienced staff to care for her, following her BMT?'

I try not to show my surprise and to let the conversation flow, continuing, 'I understand your concerns, moving from a specialist area to the adolescent unit is a big step. I'd like to reassure you that we have received a very thorough handover from the BMT team, and we will continue to work closely with them as needed.'

'Thank you, Anita, but what experience do you have of caring for children post BMT?' asks Gill.

VALUE: competence

Although I don't answer this question directly, I feel confident in my own competence, as in this unit we have had a wide range of experience caring for adolescents following BMT, and I have worked with a number of oncology patients with haematological conditions. As a team, we always endeavour to provide individualised holistic care, as we realise that all cases are individual, with unique care

MODEL: holistic care

requirements.

Instead of answering Gill, I turn to Claire: 'I'm really looking forward to getting to know you, Claire. How are you feeling today?'

Claire does not answer me but turns her head to face the window.

Gill answers instead, saying, 'Claire is reluctant to speak to people she doesn't know, so her father and I usually do this for her.'

I address Claire directly. 'That's okay Claire, I hope that over time we will get to know each other, and that you'll

VALUE: dignity and respect

feel happy to share any questions or concerns with us.'

I then explain to Claire and Gill some of the facilities on the adolescent unit, such as DVD players, computer games, table-top football, and support from a youth worker during the week. Again, I am slightly surprised by Gill's response: 'Thank you, Anita, Claire won't be needing any of those things, she likes building her Lego in her own room.'

Before I can explore more, Dr Ravi enters Claire's room, 'Good morning, Claire, Gill and Anita, how are you all this morning?'

Gill responds swiftly, 'We're okay thank you, although we were transferred to this unit unnecessarily late last night and it is quite noisy, so we have both had a disturbed night's sleep.'

At this point, Josef, Claire's dad, enters the room, breezily saying, 'Busy in here this morning, isn't it?'

'Good morning, Josef,' responds Dr Ravi. 'I have just come to say good morning to Gill and Claire and arrange to meet with you both later this morning.'

APPROACH: open communication

'Why can't we just catch up now?' Josef asks.

Dr Ravi responds warmly, 'Would you like to meet now? If so, I'll just ask one of the Clinical Nurse Specialists to join us,'

'I'm not sure I'm happy to leave Claire on her own,' says Gill hesitantly.

I step in with a solution, saying, 'I'm able to stay, if that's okay with you Claire?' Claire nods silently.

I notice Gill and Josef exchanging worried looks at this offer, but Gill agrees with what sounds like a reluctant tone, saying, 'Okay, we won't be long.'

I sit down in the chair next to Claire, where she continues to build her Lego, something I really enjoy doing with my own daughter. 'Would you like me to help you find the pieces Claire?' She nods.

For the next 15 minutes, I remain in Claire's room while her parents meet with Dr Ravi. At one point I laugh with Claire as I select the wrong piece of Lego. Claire turns to face me and smiles at my reaction to this. At this point, I know that I am beginning to build a therapeutic relationship with her

by engaging in her interests. Gill and Josef re-enter the room. Gill's face appears flushed as if she has been crying, and Josef appears stern.

'Everything okay in here?' asks Josef.

Claire nods, and I answer, 'We've been building Lego and I've been showing Claire how bad I am at finding the right pieces in the tub. I'm going to start preparing your morning medications, how do you usually like to take these Claire.

Do you like a particular drink or something to eat with them?'.

Gill answers abruptly, 'You don't need to worry. I'll sort that, just bring the meds.'

Time for bed

I hand over to Tom for the night shift. I share that Claire has had blood taken during the day shift, which shows a further increase in her infection markers and deterioration of her renal and liver function. Claire now appears visibly jaundiced and is experiencing pyrexial episodes with

rigours. Conversations have happened with her parents to discuss further escalation of care, and the family has agreed that it will not be in Claire's best interest to escalate to intensive care, but that Claire will continue to receive active treatment.

Night shift – Tom's perspective

I knock on Claire's side room door and wait for a response before entering. Gill and Josef are with Claire, and both acknowledge my presence. I know that they will be used to Anita, and I will have to build my own therapeutic relationship with the family.

'Good evening, my name is Tom, I'll be the nurse looking after you tonight. I understand you've been having some spikes in your temperature today, how are you feeling now?'

Gill answers for her daughter, 'Yes, today has been a tricky day, we need medications on time tonight, to ensure we get a good night's sleep, and we can keep this temperature under control. What time are they next due?'

'Let me go and get Claire's drug chart and we can have a look together.'

After going through the plan for Claire for the night with mum, ensuring there is appropriate time in between care rounds for Claire to get some quality sleep, Claire and her mother settle down to sleep at around ten o'clock after I complete her observations.

APPROACH: *clustering care*

At two in the morning, I enter the room where both Claire and Gill are asleep to complete physiological observations. I notice that Claire is visibly shaking with goose pimples over her skin; her skin is also hot to touch with a rising temperature. Claire wakes up while I am taking her temperature and appears visibly scared.

'Hi Claire, it's just me Tom. I'm just checking your temperature, and I can see that you're shaking. How are you feeling?'

Claire looks at me with wide scared eyes, whispering, 'Am I going to die?'

I am quite surprised by this question and, for a few seconds, am at a loss as to what to say. I take a deep breath and ask Claire, 'Why do you think you're going to die?' She replies, wide-eyed, 'Because it feels like I'm going to die right now!'

THEORY: *the 5 Ps of discussing a poor prognosis*

I am balanced with my response as I start to frame what might be the beginnings of a difficult conversation. 'You have a temperature and you're shaking because your body is trying to make your body warmer. This is caused by the infection you have, and that can feel really horrible and scary. I'm going to get you some medicine which will help bring your temperature down and stop the shaking. Would you like me to wake up your mum?'.

APPROACH: psychological and emotional support

Claire answers, 'Yes please,' so I gently walk over and wake up mum, saying, 'Gill, sorry to wake you. but Claire's got a high temperature and she's shaking. I think she's feeling a bit scared.'

Gill gets up immediately and comes to sit on the bed with Claire, who is visibly upset. She asks her mum, 'Am I going to die?' At this point, Gill looks at me with a scared expression and then turns back to her daughter and says, 'You've just got a temperature; it's all going to be okay; Tom is going to get you some medicine now.'

I leave the room and go to get medication to help stop the rigours and make her feel more comfortable. I also contact the on-call doctor to update them and they confirm the medication required and say they will be available to review her in a short while, asking me to let them know if she deteriorates further.

APPROACH: teamwork

When I return to the room, Claire is still visibly upset, and her mum is comforting her. I administer the medication and ask if there is anything else that they need at this time, reassuring them that I will be back to recheck her observations.

Half an hour later, Claire has stopped shaking and is more settled. Mum comes out of the room and again appears distressed. I ask her if she is okay. Gill says, 'I can't believe she asked me that. You have to understand I don't want her to be scared. If she knows that the treatment hasn't worked, she will be scared. I don't want her to know that we're here for palliative care.'

VALUE: self-awareness

VALUE: compassion

I am unsure how to proceed, but answer, 'I can see that you love your daughter very much, I know that you're in a really difficult situation right now, which is distressing for all of you. I also understand, why you would want to protect her and help her not feel scared.'

I pause here to observe Gill's reaction. She seems receptive to what I am saying, so I continue, 'I wonder whether she is already scared because she doesn't really understand what's going on in her body. And maybe having some knowledge of that might help her feel less scared. Knowing that you are there definitely makes her feel safe and that's what she wanted when she woke up. She was clearly scared and wanted me to wake you.'

APPROACH: advocating for autonomy

Gill responds by asking abruptly, 'So you think I should have told her right now, in the middle of the night, that she's going to die and that she's on end-of-life care?'

I feel like I am being drawn into a bit of a trap. 'The middle of the night when she's scared because she has a fever is probably not the best time to have that conversation. But the fact she asked whether she is going to die shows that she has questions and is thinking she might die.' I pause at this point to gauge how Gill is receiving this information. Her body language appears more open, so I continue, 'I wonder if a good time would be when you and her dad are both here, as well as a consultant and the nurse specialist who can be available to answer any questions that she might have. We wouldn't expect parents to talk to their children on their own about this. It is such a difficult thing even for health professionals to talk about.'

VALUE: compassion

MODEL: family-centred care

Gill seems to take this information on board. She then turns to me and says, 'I think you're right that now is not the right time. I'm going to try and get a few more hours sleep. Thank you for your help with Claire tonight. Will you let me know if she has another fever?'

To which I reply, 'Yes, of course I will.'

I document our conversation in the patient's notes so that the medical and nursing team will be able to continue the discussion and be prepared that Claire is starting to explore her prognosis. By three o'clock, Claire has gone back to sleep and is settled. She has no further high fever spikes. She has blood tests taken at 6 am, and the only ongoing

APPROACH: teamwork

issues are a low-grade fever and a mild tachycardia. The remainder of my shift is quiet.

At the morning handover, Anita is taking over from me, as she is doing two long days in a row and is going to be following on with Claire's care. It makes handover easier, as I explain what happened overnight. Anita thinks this is a big step for Gill. She reassures me that she will share my discussions and highlight this to the medical team and nurse specialist so that they can follow this up with Gill and Josef today.

APPROACH: continuity of care

Day shift 2 – Anita's perspective

After receiving my initial handover from Tom, I review the notes that he has written from the previous night's conversation, as well as the observations and changes to Claire's medication. At 8 am, I go in to check on Claire, who is not yet awake. Mum is also asleep still, so I leave them to rest. At nine o'clock, I take in Claire's morning oral medication, and they are both awake. Claire acknowledges me with a smile, which feels like good progress from the previous day's lack of eye contact. Gill also seems genuinely relieved to see me, as she says, 'Oh good, it's you, Anita. I won't have to explain everything again to another new nurse, we have a busy day ahead of us.'

APPROACH: continuity of care

To which Claire asks, 'Busy, how mum?'

'You know Reverend Dominic is coming in today for your baptism, remember we discussed this before we left the BMT unit.'

Claire replies in a non-committal tone, 'Oh yeah, okay.'

Gill rejoins with enthusiasm, 'Anita I'm not sure if I told you yesterday but he's coming around midday and we would really like Claire to be off her Intravenous lines at the time of the baptism.'

I say, 'Oh, I'm sure we can work around that. How long do you think the baptism will take?'

'Oh, no more than 20 minutes, I'm sure,' Gill replies, adding, 'In fact, it would be really useful if you and maybe Hannah the nurse specialist could be here at the time, as I believe there need to be witnesses – a bit like a wedding maybe.' Gill laughs quietly at her own joke.

Claire does not see the humour in this and frowns at her mum saying, 'Oh I don't want it to be a big deal, you promised lots of people wouldn't need to be involved.'

Gill answers, 'No there won't be lots of people – just you, me your dad and two nurses. That's hardly many people.'

Claire makes a non-committal sound and goes back to playing on her phone.

Gill turns to her, saying, 'Come on, you know we discussed this.' Claire only nods at her mum.

Gill then asks me, 'Do you think you will be allowed to be available at midday?'

I am not a Christian, so I feel uncomfortable at this request to be involved. 'Thank you for asking me and I would be happy to be a witness if I can be spared from my other patient duties. I will check with the nurse in charge whether someone can cover for me. However, I should let you know that I'm not a Christian and don't have any specific affiliation to any faith. But if that is okay with you then I am happy to be a witness.'

APPROACH: *spiritual care*

Gill says, 'Oh that's absolutely fine, my husband doesn't believe but understands how important this is for me and Claire. I hope the nurse in charge can find cover.' Gill leaves the room to make her breakfast, and I ask Claire, 'How are you feeling this morning? Tom your nurse last night told me about your fever in the night.'

APPROACH: *advocating for autonomy*

Claire looks at me, shrugs her shoulders, and goes back to her phone. I ask her if I can check her temperature now, and she agrees. Her mum comes back in while I am doing the observations and asks what her temperature is. At 37.7, it is the lowest it has been for the last 12 hours.

When the medical team and nurse specialist arrived for the ward round, they informed me that Claire's liver and renal function have deteriorated further. I let them know about the plans for the baptism today and the conversation Tom had with Gill during the night. A plan is made for the consultant and nurse specialist to sit down with Claire's mum and dad again and discuss the information Claire may need. The consultant is concerned that Claire may not be aware of the true motivation behind the hospital-based baptism and wonders if it is time to discuss advanced care planning with the family.

APPROACH: open communication

MODEL: advanced care planning in adolescents

Reflections

Anita and Tom's shared reflection: Claire's case underscored the complexity of providing care to a terminally ill adolescent within the context of family dynamics that resist sharing the terminally ill prognosis. It was pivotal when advocating for Claire's rights that we provided compassionate support to her family and ensured that Claire's remaining time is as peaceful and meaningful as possible. Through careful ethical consideration, open communication, and a commitment to holistic care, we navigated this difficult situation, balancing the needs and wishes of both Claire and her family. This case highlights critical aspects of holistic, family-centred care, compassion in end-of-life discussions, and the need for sensitivity in balancing clinical responsibilities with emotional support.

As children's and young people's nurses working with children in palliative care, it is essential to encompass key skills such as empathy, adaptability, collaboration, and patient-family advocacy. By carefully balancing the medical and emotional needs of the patient and her family, we were able to provide a nuanced and empathetic approach to care during an emotionally charged time.

Anita's reflection: The initial interaction with Claire's mother shows a challenging but necessary rapport-building phase (Quinn, 2022). Gill's concern over my nursing experience and expertise reflects understandable anxiety, as

Claire has moved from a specialist unit to a general adolescent ward, intensifying Gill's fears about the quality of care. By acknowledging Gill's concerns, maintaining open communication, and providing reassurance about continuity of care from the BMT team, I was able to demonstrate a family-centred care approach to relationship building. To build trust with Claire's family, which is crucial given the emotional weight they carried, I started by establishing a relationship based on transparency and empathy.

The interaction around Claire's baptism presented an ethical and emotional aspect of care. While remaining professional and expressing no affiliation with a faith, I was able to demonstrate a respect for their family's beliefs and wishes. A willingness to be involved in the baptism, contingent on covering nursing responsibilities, exemplifies my accommodating, supportive stance, which is vital for respecting family-centred care and supporting spiritual needs.

Tom's reflection: Attending to Claire's physical and emotional needs during her night-time febrile episode demonstrated adaptability and sensitivity to the current situation. Claire's question about death signalled her awareness of her declining condition, although she may have lacked the context to fully comprehend it. Responding to her question by explaining her symptoms while assessing her readiness for further information reflected my compassionate approach to addressing a challenging existential inquiry. Recognising the family's protective stance, it was still important to suggest to Gill the importance of openness in addressing Claire's fears. This interaction underscored my role as a nurse in advocating and using clear communication while providing sensitive, age-appropriate information that empowers patients and helps them cope with their health journey.

The shift from curative to palliative care planning is a delicate transition, requiring the involvement of a multidisciplinary team. To maintain a compassionate and sensitive approach to end-of-life care, I used open communication with Gill about Claire's prognosis while considering Claire's readiness to hear the truth. Documenting these interactions further emphasises the importance of continuity in communication among caregivers and the multidisciplinary teams when managing this transition.

Questions for reflection and discussion

Explore the key issues raised in the above scenario as you answer the following six questions:

1. What steps could be taken to further support a family in their emotional journey as they come to terms with the prognosis of their child or adolescent?

2. How can health professionals maintain empathy and professionalism when families like Claire's are resistant to certain medical recommendations, such as transitioning to palliative care?

3. How should nurses collaborate with other members of the healthcare team to address both Claire's clinical needs and her family's reluctance to discuss end-of-life care?

4. How can nurses tailor their care to fit their patients' interests, personality, and emotional needs?

5. How might dealing with end-of-life care for young patients impact health practitioners emotionally and mentally? What self-care or professional support strategies could help with managing the emotional demands of such cases?

6. How could Anita's approach to supporting the family's desire for Claire's baptism reflect a broader understanding of spiritual care, even when she expresses no personal religious affiliation?

Further reading

European Association for Palliative Care (2022) *European Charter on Palliative Care for Children and Young People*. https://eapcnet.eu/eapc-groups/reference/children-young-people/

Kaye, E.C., Woods, C., Kennedy, K., Velrajan, S., Gattas, M., Bilbeisi, T., Huber, R., Lemmon, M.E., Baker, J.N., and Mack, J.M. (2021) Communication around palliative care principles and advance care planning between oncologists, children with advancing cancer and families. *British Journal of Cancer*, 125: 1089–1099 https://doi.org/10.1038/s41416-021-01512-9

NHS Golden Jubilee (2023) *Spiritual Care Strategy* 2023–2026. https://www.nhsgoldenjubilee.co.uk/application/files/6816/6936/7153/Spiritual_Care_Strategy_2023.pdf

Turnbull, C. (2024) Navigating the shift from curative treatment in palliative care: Advice for nurses on communicating bad news to patients, supporting them in advanced stages of illness and explaining what palliative care is. *Cancer Nursing Practice*, 23(2): 7–9. doi:10.7748/cnp.23.2.7. s3.

Universal Principles for Advance Care Planning https://www.england.nhs.uk/wp-content/uploads/2022/03/universal-principles-for-advance-care-planning.pdf

Further information

VALUES

Compassion in palliative care is essential to supporting care needs and is characterised by a deep sense of understanding, concern, and a proactive desire to alleviate the suffering of patients facing serious or terminal illnesses. It involves not only recognising the pain and emotional distress of patients and their families but also taking clear steps to provide comfort, dignity, and holistic support.

Dignity and respect involve honouring patients' individual needs, values, and preferences, regardless of their condition or prognosis. These values emphasise creating an environment where adolescents feel valued and are treated as unique individuals.

Self-awareness is a critical skill for nurses, especially when providing palliative care to adolescents. It involves having a deep understanding of one's own thoughts, emotions, biases, and behaviours. In the context of adolescent palliative care, self-awareness enables nurses to offer compassionate, family-centred care while navigating the complex emotional and ethical challenges that arise.

THEORIES

The 5 Ps of discussing a poor prognosis relate to how to respond to an ICU patient asking if she/he is going to die. The first P is perspective. When a patient asks, 'Am I going to die?', an effective response from the health professional is to explore the experiences and perspective of the patient asking the question, as this question is often the reflection of other unspoken concerns the patient has, which can originate from fear, pain, physical suffering, and existential and spiritual distress. Understanding the perspective of the patient at this moment will ensure that the health professional addresses the specific concern (Isaac and Curtis, 2017).

Transactional Model of Communication: Barnlund (1970) views communication as a dynamic, interactive process where both parties influence each other. It highlights the importance of feedback, context, and the ongoing nature of communication and focuses on engaging in two-way communication with adolescents, actively seeking their input and responding to their feedback. The theory encourages the avoidance of one-sided conversations where only the adult is speaking and advises paying attention to non-verbal cues, such as body language and facial expressions. These are particularly important in understanding adolescents who may struggle to articulate their feelings verbally.

APPROACHES

Advocating for autonomy in adolescent palliative care, advocating for autonomy means respecting the young person's voice and choices, even when they are facing serious or life-limiting illness. This approach acknowledges the evolving capacity of adolescents to understand their situation, make decisions, and express preferences about their treatment and quality of life.

Clustering care refers to performing multiple care activities at once instead of spreading them throughout the night shift, meaning that patients experience fewer interruptions to their sleep, leading to better quality rest. Minimising the number of times a patient is woken up for procedures reduces stress and discomfort, enhancing their overall experience. Adequate sleep is crucial for healing and recovery, so clustering care can positively impact patient outcomes. There needs to be careful evaluation of each patient's individual needs to determine the optimal timing for clustered care, with willingness to adjust the clustering schedule based on patient needs and unexpected situations.

Continuity of care provides a seamless and coordinated experience for young patients as they move through different phases of their illness and interact with various healthcare providers. This type of continuity ensures that the patient and their family receive consistent, comprehensive, and personalised care throughout their entire journey. Adolescents benefit from building trusting relationships with a consistent team of healthcare practitioners. Continuity means minimising the number of different nurses involved in their care. This approach helps the adolescent feel secure and understood as they develop rapport with nurses who are familiar with their preferences, needs, and personal history.

Open communication between medical teams and parents who are hesitant to tell their adolescent about a terminal prognosis is essential for building trust, guiding decision-making, and ensuring the best possible care for the adolescent. It allows for a compassionate, supportive approach that respects both the parents' fears and the adolescent's right to information. Open communication can help uncover the underlying reasons why parents may not want to tell their adolescents about the prognosis. These reasons can include fear of causing emotional distress, cultural beliefs, denial, or a desire to maintain hope.

Psychological and emotional support is essential in adolescence, which is a time of exploring identity and seeking independence. An illness may disrupt the process of identity formation, causing frustration or a sense of lost autonomy. Nurses can support the adolescent by encouraging participation in decision-making and validating their feelings. Providing tools for coping, like mindfulness techniques, journaling, or art therapy, can help adolescents express their emotions and reduce stress.

Spiritual care involves understanding and respecting the adolescent's cultural background and personal values and is critical to providing emotional support that aligns with their beliefs. Adolescents may grapple with questions about the meaning of life, their purpose and what comes after death. Spiritual care providers, such as hospital chaplains or spiritual counsellors, can help explore these questions, regardless of the adolescent's religious or spiritual beliefs.

Teamwork is a vital aspect of adolescent palliative care, ensuring that comprehensive and coordinated care is delivered to meet the complex needs of a young person. In palliative care, the nursing team often collaborates with a broader multidisciplinary team, but the cohesion and collaboration between nursing staff are crucial for high-quality care. Effective communication is essential within teamwork, as nurses need to share information accurately and in a timely manner to ensure seamless care. Clear documentation and communication systems help prevent misunderstandings and ensure that all team members have access to the most up-to-date information about the adolescent's condition.

MODELS

Advanced care planning in adolescents is a proactive process of discussing and documenting preferences for future healthcare in situations where the young persons might be unable to make decisions themselves due to illness or incapacity. This process is particularly important for adolescents living with serious, chronic, or life-limiting conditions.

Family-centred care respects the cultural and family network of the adolescent, ensuring that both the patient and family members receive guidance and emotional support.

Holistic care in adolescent palliative care is an approach that aims to address the complete spectrum of needs – physical, emotional, social, and spiritual – of adolescents facing serious, life-limiting illnesses. The goal is to enhance the quality of life for both the adolescent and their family, recognising the unique developmental stage and challenges of adolescence.

References

Barnlund, D.C. (1970). A transactional model of communication. In Akin, J., Goldberg, A., Stewart, J. and Myers, G. (eds.), Language behavior: A book of readings in communication, 43–61. The Hague: Mouton. 10.1515/9783110878752.43

Isaac, M. and Curtis, R. (2017) How to respond to an ICU patient asking if she/he is going to die. *Intensive Care Med*, 43(2): 220–222. doi: 10.1007/s00134-016-4533-y.

Quinn, H. (2022) Why rapport matters: Building the nurse-patient relationship. *Nursing Standard*, 37(8): 39–42. doi: 10.7748/ns.37.8.39. S17.

Case study 5
Lily: in whose best interests?

Kirsty Henry and Christine Nightingale

'You have a new message'

Lily's mum left a voice message on the out-of-hours phone system. Her daughter has just received an invitation to attend for cervical screening at her local GP clinic. Lily will be 25 in a few months' time and will reach the age to be included in the UK national cervical screening programme (NHS, 2024a). I have had contact with Lily for the past 6 years as her Community Learning Disability Nurse (CLDN) and have met her mum on a couple of occasions. Although my role is supporting the healthcare needs of children and adults with an intellectual disability, in practice this is often undertaken with the support of family members and carers. I recognise that Lily's mum will be worried by the invitation for cervical screening, and she may be wondering whether Lily should have this procedure. Lily is her only child, born prematurely, with a long and traumatic delivery for both herself and her mother. Lily did not meet her developmental milestones and was diagnosed with a 'mild to moderate' intellectual disability.

THEORY: NHS cervical screening strategy

THEORY: intellectual disability

Lily is an outgoing young woman who is attending college and learning kitchen skills. She is an enthusiastic student, always willing to participate in the tasks set by her tutors. Her receptive language skills are good, and she follows instructions in the training kitchen well if these are given in short sentences. However, she finds it difficult to understand abstract and complex ideas and prefers longer instructions to be augmented with pictorial or 'easy read' pictures and symbols, supported with sign language. She has a great desire to please others and will pick up on speech prosody and intonational cues, where the speaker places stress on particular words or phrases to convey a specific meaning or bias. Lily's verbal or expressive skills are more limited. She sometimes feels challenged in constructing more complex sentences and will often resort

APPROACH: augmentative and alternative communication

DOI: 10.4324/9781003651758-5

to short responses and sign language, only expanding her answers if skilfully prompted. Popular with her peer group, Lily is very happy at college and has been going out for evenings with her friends to the pubs and nightclubs, much to her mum's alarm.

Preparation for an episode of care with Lily

Last year, I completed the assessments within the Moulster and Griffiths Learning Disability Nursing model (Atkinson et al., 2016; Moulster et al., 2019), which identified Lily's health and social risks as well as her future wishes. I concluded that whilst Lily had reasonably good support from education, health, and social care services, her communication and cognitive processing skills, along with difficulties in accessing services independently, mean that she is at moderate risk of experiencing significant health inequalities in her lifetime. Lily's risk of cervical cancer was assessed to be slightly elevated because mum had not given consent for Lily to have the Human Papilloma Virus (HPV) vaccination when she was a teenager.

MODEL: person-centred practice

THEORY: health inequalities

Lily and I used the 'Person Centred Screening Tool' (Moulster et al., 2019) to map out her future life and care goals. Lily made it clear that she wants to attend all her relevant healthcare appointments, just like her friends at college. I was really pleased that she was keen to have her health screening but was not entirely confident that Lily understood health screening procedures sufficiently to give an informed choice. At the time, Lily had been quite giggly when talking about boyfriends. She had her eye on one of the lads on the catering course. Fortunately, her college had received funding to design and deliver sex education and safer sex courses, and Lily was on this programme, so I did not take any further action at that time.

THEORY: informed choice

I am in no doubt that Lily should now be supported to make an informed choice about whether to go forward for a cervical screening appointment. I am working collaboratively with Jak, the GP nurse practitioner. As a CLDN, it is

MODEL: nursing assessment

APPROACH: multi-professional working

not within my job role to perform cervical screening but instead to facilitate access to mainstream services where possible. Jak is an experienced practice nurse who has supported many women and people with a cervix on their first procedures. Jak, the GP surgery's nurse practitioner, is anxious about taking a cervical cellular sample from a woman who has limited verbal communication skills and who may lack the capacity to fully understand the invasive nature of the procedure. Our dilemma is that whilst Lily is keen to engage in a cervical examination, this willingness is based on her desire to be like her friends and possibly to please me. Willingness to engage does not equate to consent to the procedure. The first principle of the Mental Capacity Act is the presumption that an individual has the capacity to make a decision. The second principle is that an individual should be given all practical help to make an informed choice. The Mental Capacity Act (2005) is clear on the conditions for informed consent. Jak and I must be sure that Lily understands the information we give her; she can remember and weigh up the information long enough to be able to make the decision and then communicate her decision to others.

THEORY: Mental Capacity Act, 2005

Our thoughts are focused on the most effective and evidence-based ways to support Lily in gaining understanding of cervical screening. We consider what Lily might need to know about a procedure which examines internal parts of her body that she cannot see. We are also aware that whilst Lily is an adult attending sex education classes, her mum is influential and protects her from worldly information. Mum needs to be included in any plan to educate Lily on cervical screening. It is possible that Lily is now sexually active, which would raise her risk of cervical cancer. If this is so, we also need to consider whether a 'Best Interests' decision may be needed in the event that Lily is unable to make an informed choice (Mental Capacity Act, 2005).

APPROACH: evidence-based practice

APPROACH: involving and supporting family and friends

APPROACH: best interest decision

We contact Lily via a video call, saying and signing, "Hello, my name is...". Lily asks her mum to sit in on the call to help her remember what is said. We tell Lily in short sentences, supplemented with an easy-read plan, what we

APPROACH: "Hello, my name is ..." campaign

propose over the next four weeks. We agree with mum that the process of having a speculum inserted into the vagina could seem very strange to Lily, and we explain the proposed four-week plan of preparation to address

any anxieties she might have. On the call, we show Lily a sample of publications with pictorial representations of some of the stages of taking a cervical sample and an easy-read publication produced by the NHS (2024b). Lily smiles and says she wants more like that, adding that her college's assessment of her reading skills showed that she was improving and could read plain and uncomplicated texts. We agree that we will provide mum with leaflets and links with further explanations, such as those written on the NHS (2024c) cervical screening webpages.

Week one

Lily is at the door, grinning from ear to ear before I can knock. Mum hovers behind, looking slightly anxious. I feel empathy with mum and wonder whether she fears

that the process could be a physical assault on Lily. I ask Lily if she would like to share the easy-read and access-ible information Jak and I had gathered with her mum. I want to empower Lily as much as possible, reasoning that it would be a positive outcome if Lily understood the cer-

vical screening process even if she later declined to go fur-ther. As I show both women the easy-read and pictorial versions of the procedure, Lily indicates that she has seen the cross-section picture of the vagina and cervix in her classes at college. She runs to get her college folder to show us. I register mum's surprise. For me, this was good; it shows that Lily is retaining and applying information that she has previously learned. I give mum further information and links to online descriptions.

Week two

Today we meet in the clinic room at the GP surgery after

Jak has seen other patients. This visit is prearranged to avoid a long wait, which could provoke anxiety for Lily. It also means that Jak can give Lily their full attention without disrupting the appointment system. Lily has brought along her handheld device to play games or watch a video in case of a short wait. We have planned for the visit to be as informal as possible, which gives us all an opportunity to recap what Lily thinks about the information I gave her the week before. Lily points to the picture she had of the speculum and brush and says, 'Show this.' Jak asks Lily if she would like to see everything that is used during the procedure. She eagerly nods.

Jak talks Lily through the process from the point of getting onto the couch. Jak has an anatomical model of the female pelvic area and demonstrates how the sample is taken. Lily operates the lamp and looks through the open speculum, inserting the brush following Jak's instructions. Mum has a look too. Jak offers Lily the opportunity to take home a spare speculum and some brushes for a few days to look at and hold. Jak and I have previously decided not to suggest that Lily attempt inserting the brushes into her own vagina. Finally, we suggest that Lily uses a mirror to look at how her urethra, vagina, and anus are positioned.

Week three

Because Jak's work calendar was full, we agree to have a video call to check how Lily has got on with the equipment she has been lent. Lily tells us that her college friends are very jealous that she has been to the surgery and operated the examination lamp. She has also told other students in the sex education class about using a mirror to inspect themselves. Mum says they have both had a good laugh lying on their backs practising the cervical screening position with their legs apart as shown in the leaflets. Mum reports that she has asked Lily what would happen next, and Lily had correctly indicated where the speculum would be inserted in her vagina.

Jak asks Lily why she thinks smear tests are undertaken. Lily pulls a face and does a thumbs down sign, saying, 'No bad sickness.' Lily is restless, so we finish by agreeing on a further visit to the GP practice, with an opportunity for Lily to book a cervical screening appointment. Lily leaves to play a game on her handheld device. We can see that mum watches for Lily to leave the room: she wants to speak to us alone. She asks whether this is all necessary: does Lily really need this test? It is a good question. Whose best interest is served by this procedure? Mum says that, without question, Lily will give it a go, but she is concerned that the reality is far different from the theory. We agree. We assure mum that, if the screening goes ahead, Lily will be able to stop it at any point, and that the procedure will be conducted at the pace Lily dictates. Lily can bring her handheld device with her too, Jak suggests, as we close the meeting.

Week four

This is the last planned preparation or 'desensitising visit' to the GP surgery. Again, we have booked some time with Jak out of hours. Lily bounds into the room ahead of her mum. Jak shows Lily how she calls up her health records on the computer and then asks her to tell her about the cervical examination. Lily now has copies of the information on her handheld device and shows this to Jak, at the same time opening her legs and pointing to the relevant parts of her body. Jak asks, as we had before, about why people had the test. She then reminds Lily that it is not compulsory to have this done. It is her choice. Finally, Jak asks Lily if she would like to have the test herself, meaning sometime in the future. Lily verbalised and signed 'yes' and pointed to the image of a cervical screening examination in progress. She then removes the bottom layer of her clothes and positions herself on the examination couch. I catch mum's eye, and she nods. We do not need her consent, but her approval is important to Lily, Jak, and myself. Although not planned, Jak has the time, and the equipment is ready to attempt the examination. Jak reassures Lily that she can say or sign 'no' at any time to slow down or stop the procedure. Lily verbalises and nods 'yes', then starts a game on her handheld device. Jak washes her hands, slips on her gloves and begins.

Once completed, Lily says, 'Your turn now, Mum!'

Reflections

After Lily's successful cervical screening examination, I reflected on each part of the episode of care. There was no question that Lily had engaged well with the preparatory activities, including the learning objects and home and surgery visits. It dawned on me, as the anxiety of the last few weeks drained away, that I had been so keen to do a thorough job in educating and preparing Lily that I had not really listened to or heard what Lily was trying to communicate to me. With all my good intentions to 'enable' Lily to make an informed choice, I had not supported her to lead this episode of care. I had made such a big thing about cervical screening that I was in danger of prejudicing her access and entitlement to take charge of this procedure. I have thought about where my anxiety comes from. I have cervical screening myself, so I know it isn't the most pleasant or comfortable clinical procedure. Yet I have no anxieties about attending my appointments. I wondered about the social stigma directed towards cervical cancer and screening. Two studies show that negative stigma impacts women's willingness to engage in the procedure (Peterson et al., 2021; Morse et al., 2023).

THEORY: unconscious bias

I have also had conversations with practitioners skilled in taking cervical samples who said that they would absolutely refuse to undertake cervical screening with a person with an intellectual disability because it would be 'rape by speculum'. This is both an emotive and stigmatising view. I could see that I was holding within me this negative social stigma. This irrational and unconscious fear was impacting my practice. The NMC Code clearly states that nurses must, '...be aware at all times of how [y]our behaviour can affect and influence the behaviour of other people' (NMC, 2018: 20.3).

My personal lack of awareness led to me missing at least four opportunities to pick up clues that Lily understood more than I had assumed. The first opportunity was missed when Lily told me she wanted to have the same tests and health screening experiences as her peer group at college. I didn't check to understand what she already knew. The second missed opportunity was on the first visit to her home. Lily knew why I was there and what we were planning to do and was excited. I could have used her enthusiasm and motivation to find out what she needed to know, instead of ploughing on with my education plan. The third missed opportunity was our first visit to the surgery. Lily's questions were practical and about the equipment; she was clear on the process. The fourth missed opportunity was when I failed to recognise that Lily was getting bored with our cautious and slow approach (continually checking that she had understood, retained, and processed the information about cervical screening). In the middle of the video meeting, she wandered off to play on her handheld device. Lily finally took the lead, took her clothes off, and got on the couch to show us she was ready and consented to the procedure.

I was conscious of my nursing responsibility to, '...pay special attention to promoting wellbeing, preventing ill health and meeting the changing health and care needs of people during all life stages' (NMC, 2018: 3.1) against the need to 'take measures to reduce as far as possible the likelihood of mistakes, near misses, harm and the effect of harm if it takes place' (NMC, 2018: 19.1). Cervical screening is an intimate and invasive procedure; there is a clear risk of psychological harm if this procedure is not carefully explained and understood. I am pleased with the rigorous steps we took to find accessible information for Lily and the reasonable adjustments we made for her to access the GP surgery during less busy times. This plan worked well and is a potential model for interventions with other service users.

Finally, my personal and professional beliefs in promoting equity and inclusion were important at this time. I was aware that if I had done nothing to support Lily in her decision-making about cervical screening, I would be increasing the chances of her experiencing health inequalities, complex morbidity, and preventable mortality (Heslop et al., 2013; White et al., 2023).

Questions for reflection and discussion

Explore the key issues raised in the above scenario as you answer the following six questions:

1. Complete a reflection on your own thoughts and feelings about discussing an intimate procedure with someone who might have limited understanding and experience of their own body. How would you prepare for this discussion, and what would you want to know?

2. How might using a 'desensitising' approach support an individual who is anxious about a procedure, such as having an intramuscular injection at the vaccine clinic?

3. Find two or three patient information leaflets. These might be about a specific long-term health condition, how to apply or take prescribed medications, or how to apply for benefits or care support. Using the Cabinet Office (2024) guidance on plain English, assess whether the leaflets you have chosen could be improved.

4. Search, find and practise the signs for 'hello, my name is …' and for 'yes' and 'no.' Reflect on how the use of basic sign language can contribute to a reduction in health inequalities and diagnostic overshadowing.

5. How could encouraging and supporting people with a learning disability to attend screening impact on the length and quality of their lives?

6. What other parts of the NMC (2018) Code could be applied to the reflection on this episode of care?

Further reading

Baines, S., Emerson, E., Robertson, J. and Hatton, C. (2018) Sexual activity and sexual health among young adults with and without mild/moderate intellectual disability. *BMC Public Health* 18: 667. https://doi.org/10.1186/s12889-018-5572-9

Hollins, S., Downer, J. and Bailey, H. (2024) Keeping Healthy Down Below, Books Beyond Words, https://booksbeyondwords.co.uk/bookshop/paperbacks/keeping-healthy-down-below

Malik, R. (2023) Supporting people with learning disabilities to have blood tests, *Learning Disability Practice*, 23(1): 18–25. doi: 10.7748/ld. 2020.e2023.

Mencap (2024) Information about cervical screening. https://www.mencap.org.uk/easyread/information-about-cervical-screening-test (Accessed 1st September 2024).

Mencap (2024) Tips for good communication. https://www.mencap.org.uk/easyread/tips-good-communication (Accessed 1st September 2024).

Further information

VALUES

Empathy is the ability to take on the perspective of others and understand what they may be feeling.

Empowerment enables people to make choices and decisions about their own lives by involving them in the design of their care and support.

THEORIES

Health inequalities refer to avoidable differences in health outcomes, noticeable across different groups in society.

Informed choice: For a person to consent to treatment or a procedure, or to deny consent, they must be given all the information about that treatment or procedure, including potential benefits, side effects, alternatives, and consequences of not undergoing treatment. However, it is not sufficient to simply provide information; clinicians must ensure that the information is accessible to the person to enable them to make an informed decision. This may involve adjustments to language, settings, text information, or the use of alternative formats, including Easy Read information.

Intellectual disability and learning disability are used interchangeably within the UK. In England and Wales, the term learning disability is generally adopted, whilst internationally, the term intellectual disability is preferred.

Mental Capacity Act (2005) provides a legislative framework to support decision-making for people aged 16 and over in England and Wales. It establishes five principles, including the presumption of capacity, clarifies a four-stage test to assess capacity, and provides a clear process of decision-making when a person is assessed to lack the capacity to make a specific decision.

NHS Cervical Cancer Strategy relates to the NHS (2023) pledge to eliminate cervical cancer by 2040 through a two-pronged approach – firstly, getting everyone vaccinated against HPV and then, for people with a cervix, to be tested for the presence of HPV and, if needed, a further examination of cervical cells for pre-cancerous and cancerous changes.

Unconscious bias in learning disability care acknowledges that whilst clinical decisions are made with the best of intentions, based on knowledge, skill, and experience, we also need to be aware that decision-making can be influenced by a practitioner's perception of the patient's inability to cope with or consent to treatment or by assumptions around a person's quality of life (White et al., 2023).

APPROACHES

"Hello, my name is …" campaign was founded by Dr Kate Granger prior to her death in 2016. As a patient with terminal cancer, Kate identified what she described as a 'stark reality' that clinicians were failing to introduce themselves before delivering care. As a clinician, Kate understood the importance of communication in the delivery of compassionate healthcare. The campaign has four key values: Communication, The Little Things, Patients at the Heart of all Decisions, and See Me. More information on Kate's campaign and legacy, alongside these core values, can be found at https://www.hellomynameis.org.uk/

Augmentative and Alternative Communication (AAC) incorporates a wide range of techniques that support (augment) or replace spoken communication. These include 'no-tech' means such as gestures, body language, and sign-language; 'low-tech' means such as objects of reference and pictures like Easy Read; and 'high tech' means which include tablets, electronic communication boards, and Voice Output Communication Aids (VOCAs). AACs enable communication to be as effective as possible.

Best interest decision is the process of determining the outcome of a decision that is in a person's best interests where they are assessed as lacking the capacity to make that decision under the Mental Capacity Act (2005).

Desensitisation is a process used to reduce an emotional response, such as anxiety or fear, to a particular stimulus by gradual or repeated exposure.

Evidence-based practice involves using the best available evidence from reliable sources to plan and deliver care.

Multi-professional working is where people from more than one professional discipline work together to achieve the best outcomes for the patient. In intellectual disability practice, this may include health and social care professionals working alongside private and voluntary sector workers and advocacy services. To ensure a seamless and cohesive service, clear and timely communication between professionals is key. A good understanding of each other's roles is essential to effective interprofessional working.

Involving and supporting family and friends recognises that effective care is not just for the person who is ill but for all the people who are important in their life. People with an intellectual disability may have different social networks than those in the general population, including close relationships with parents, siblings, friends, and carers. It is important to establish who is important to that person and ensure that they are involved as partners in care and offered support.

Person-centred practice within intellectual disability practice includes considering a person's capacity, their communication needs and the role of formal and informal caregivers (Moulster et al., 2019).

Reasonable adjustments are a requirement under the Equality Act (2010) to enable people with protected characteristics, including but not restricted to people with a disability, to be able to access and receive equitable services.

MODELS

Nursing assessment is an ongoing and comprehensive evaluation of the psychological, social, and physical well-being by nurses of individuals in their care.

Reflection in action is a process of analysing practice, thoughts, feelings, and values as practitioners go about their work.

References

Atkinson, D., Boulter, P., Hebron, C. and Moulster, G. (2013) *The Health Equalities Framework (HEF): An outcomes framework based on the determinants of health inequalities*. UK Learning Disability Consultant Nurse Network. Available at: https://www.debramooreassociates.com/hef (Accessed 3rd February 2025).

Cabinet Office (2024) Functional standards writing style guide, https://www.gov.uk/government/publications/handbook-for-standard-managers/functional-standards-writing-style-guide (Accessed 10th September 2024).

Equality Act (2010) c. 15. Available at: https://www.legislation.gov.uk/ukpga/2010/15 (Accessed 31st January 2025).

Heslop, P., Blair, P., Fleming, P., Hoghton, M., Marriott, A. and Russ, L. (2013) *Confidential Inquiry into Premature Deaths of People with Learning Disabilities (CIPOLD)*. Bristol, Norah Fry Research Centre.

Mental Capacity Act (2005) c. 9. Available at: https://www.legislation.gov.uk/ukpga/2005/9/contents/enacted (Accessed 31st January 2025).

Morse, R.M., Brown, J., Gage, J.C., Prieto, B.A., Jurszuk, M., Matos, A., Vasquez, J., Reategui, R.R., Meza-Sanchez, L., Gravitt, P.E., Tracy, J.K., Paz-Soldan, V.A. and the Provecto Precancer Study Group (2023) "Easy women get it": Pre-existing stigma associated with HPV and cervical cancer in a low-resource setting prior to implementation of an HPV screen-and-treat program. *BMC Public Health* 23: 2396. https://doi.org/10.1186/s12889-023-17324-w (Accessed: 6th October 2024).

Moulster, G., Iorizzo, J., Ames, S. and Kernohan, J. (2019) *The Moulster and Griffiths Learning Disability Nursing Model*, London, Jessica Kingsley.

NHS (2023) NHS sets ambition to eliminate cervical cancer by 2040, https://www.england.nhs.uk/2023/11/nhs-sets-ambition-to-eliminate-cervical-cancer-by-2040/#:~:text=The%20NHS%20will%20today%20pledge,lives%20every%20year%20in%20England. (Accessed 3rd September 2024).

NHS (2024a) Cervical Screening, https://www.gov.uk/guidance/cervical-screening-programme-overview (Accessed 1st October 2024).

NHS (2024b) Having Cervical Screening, https://www.gov.uk/government/publications/cervical-screening-easy-read-guide (Accessed 1st October 2024).

NHS (2024c) Cervical Screening, https://www.nhs.uk/conditions/cervical-screening/ (Assessed 3rd September 2024).

Nursing and Midwifery Council (2018) *The Code: Professional Standards of Practice and Behaviour for Nurses, Midwives and Nursing Associates*. London, NMC.

Peterson, C., Silva, A., Goben, A.H., Ongtengco, N.P., Hu, E.Z., Khanna, D., Nussbaum, E.R., Jasenof, I.G., Kim, S.J. and Dykens, J.A (2021) Stigma and cervical cancer prevention: A scoping review of the U.S. literature. *Preventive Medicine*, 153, https://doi.org/10.1016/j.ypmed.2021.106849. (Accessed: 6th October 2024).

White, A., Sheehan, R., Ding, J., Roberts, C., Magill, N., Keagan-Bull, R., Carter, B., Chauhan, U., Tuffrey-Wijne, I. and Strydom, A. (2023) Learning from lives and deaths – people with a learning disability and autistic people (Leder) report for 2022. London, King's College London.

Case study 6
Erica: a blessing or a curse

Sarah Housden and Jayne Needham

An appointment with Erica

As a registered midwife, I can find myself working with people at times of utmost joy as well as of utter tragedy. The profound sense of awe experienced at all the potential held within new life as a person comes into the world is what first attracted me to the profession, although these days, I probably gain the greatest satisfaction from using my advanced communication and problem-solving skills in complex situations.

THEORY: emotional labour in healthcare

It has been three weeks since I last met with Erica. She is now 15 weeks pregnant, having presented with vaginal bleeding at 12 weeks. An examination at that point led to a suspicion of some abnormal cells on her cervix, for which she was referred for further exploration. At 35 years old, she has now been diagnosed with cervical cancer.

I have arranged to meet with Erica at her local community clinic in the hope that a slightly less busy environment will give her the opportunity she needs to talk through the essential issues going forward. I am particularly keen that the termination of pregnancy should take place sooner rather than later, partly in the hope of reducing the trauma Erica is likely to go through by continuing to carry an unborn child whom she is unlikely to bear to full term.

An assumption too far

'Thank you for meeting with me today, Erica,' I begin. Erica gives me a lopsided smile which betrays her efforts to keep up a brave face, despite the sadness she is experiencing.

'Shall we start with you telling me what's happened since we last met?' I suggest.

Erica averts her gaze to the side, avoiding eye contact. She begins to speak hesitantly: 'As you know Elise, I'm 35, no

DOI: 10.4324/9781003651758-6

spring chicken and this is my first pregnancy. Terry and I have been through two rounds of IVF to be able to get to this point of expecting our first child. We have been trying for a baby for ten years, and the new hope that conceiving has brought us has refreshed out marriage after so many years of disappointment and shame.'

THEORY: social stigma

She pauses and turns to look at me directly, stating in a firmer voice, 'Do you have any idea of the stigma I live with for not having any children? It's not just Terry's Mum and my Mum, asking why we don't start planning a family, but our wider family and most of our friends as well. Everyone expects us to have children, and it's what we want too.'

THEORY: social norms

As Erica speaks, I realise that I have gone too far in my assumptions and that while my personal choice in this situation would be to terminate the pregnancy to focus on my own cancer treatment, this may not be everybody's choice.

APPROACH: avoid making assumptions

VALUE: respect

'Have you been able to discuss this with anyone, Erica? What does Terry think?' I ask, wondering whether she will have proper psychological and emotional support through the decision-making process.

VALUE: compassion

MODEL: non-verbal communication

With her gaze averted again, Erica continues to share her perspective with me: 'No, to be honest, I haven't. Terry and I were going to tell everyone about the pregnancy after my last visit to you, but for the time being I have persuaded him to keep it as a surprise.' She pauses, then hesitantly tells me, 'Elise, you see, I haven't told Terry about the bleeding, or the tests, or the appointment with oncology, or even that I'm here today. I don't want him to have to choose between me and his child; I want to make that choice for him. To give him the child he so much wants.'

I feel concerned and a bit shocked about Erica making this decision alone and wonder what Terry and the wider family would actually think. I am determined to understand Erica's perspective better, though, and to try to see things from her point of view. 'Can you tell me more about what's brought you to that decision Erica?' I ask. She is silent for a few

VALUE: care

APPROACH: empathy

moments, and I remind myself that one of the skills of active listening is to allow silences to happen, even though they may feel uncomfortable.

APPROACH: active listening

A woman protects her unborn child

'I have been looking at what it says online about cancer treatments during pregnancy. From what I can gather, there is a high chance that many of the currently available treatments for Stage 2 cervical cancer might harm my unborn child. I don't want that, Elise! I have wanted and loved this baby since before the conception, and the idea of terminating the life of a wanted baby just doesn't sit at all well with me. Can you understand that?'

THEORY: digital health literacy

MODEL: stages of cervical cancer

APPROACH: human rights

I am in my mid-twenties, and there are years ahead of me when I will be able to choose to have a family or not. I am not sure that I can easily put myself in the shoes of someone who knows that the time in which to make this choice is running out. Having had some hope, only to lose that hope, must feel like an absolute tragedy.

APPROACH: lifespan approach

'I'm not in your position, Erica, but I can see that you feel strongly about this. How about we look at what can be done? Whether there are any other options; something between a termination, which you don't want, and some of the treatments for cervical cancer at this stage, which might harm your unborn child? I'm not saying for certain that there will be other options, but I do hear what you are saying and that you don't want to have a termination. I want to reassure you that nothing will happen without your consent. That whatever I, Terry, or the consultant oncologist thinks, we are going to look together at all the possible options before coming to a conclusion about the best course of action. Now tell me, what has the oncologist suggested treatment wise, or have you not had that conversation yet?'

APPROACH: recognising feelings

APPROACH: validation

VALUE: consent

APPROACH: shared decision-making

A new perspective

'I'm not religious you know, and never have been,' Erica says unexpectedly, her voice softening and her body visibly relaxing. 'It's not that I have a strong view about pregnancy termination usually, at all. It's just that I feel like there is a precious life in me, that is part of me, that represents my hopes for the future – not just for me and Terry, but a wider kind of hope that extends beyond our lives. I think I've become very protective of this life within me that represents that hope, and I feel like I've got to protect this life even if it means losing my own. I don't know where these thoughts and feelings have come from because I've not had any particular religious or even philosophical thoughts prior to becoming pregnant. It's as though it has changed something within me. But now I feel like this life has been entrusted to me, and that I have a responsibility to sustain it, whatever the cost.'

VALUE: Hope

I smile warmly at Erica, recognising echoes of what I've heard from other women in some of what she says. 'There is certainly something different that happens when someone is expecting a baby,' I say, thinking to myself that while it is not a universal experience, it is real for many women. I wonder whether it is changes in hormones or maybe some other aspect of the experience which can open a woman's eyes to a different side of themselves and to the meaning of life when they are expecting a baby.

MODEL: person-centred practice

VALUE: curiosity

Finding a way forward

I had started the appointment thinking that we would be organising a termination as swiftly as possible. Now, while keeping a potential termination as a secondary thought which may need action in a few weeks, I am turning my thinking towards the availability of more conservative, or delayed, treatments for the cervical cancer.

APPROACH: patient-centred goal planning

'I shall write to your oncologist today and request a review of treatment options,' I tell Erica, going on to explain, 'We do need to keep our minds open to making difficult choices along the way, but I want you to know that I will walk this path with you, as far as my professional role enables me to'.

APPROACH: teamwork

'Thank you, Elise. I thought everyone would be convinced I should have a termination and would stop me from trying to save my unborn child, but it really feels like you have listened to me. It was such a blessing when the IVF finally worked, and I have felt mentally tortured at the prospect of losing this baby. It was like a blessing being turned into a curse when I found out about the cancer. I just can't explain the turmoil I've been going through.'

'Before we finish for today, Erica, would you feel able to speak with Terry about the cancer now? You really need someone who can support you in making decisions for your own good, as well as for your unborn child'.

THEORY: emotional support

Erica hesitates before replying, 'Yes, Elise, I'll speak to him today. No point in delaying the inevitable any further.'

Reflections

One of my greatest concerns in looking back at this inter-action with Erica was whether I was giving her false hope or even avoiding an emotionally conflictual conversation due to not wanting to break bad news or reinforce the bad news that she has already heard. Alternatively, there is great sense in this approach, as I am working with the indi-vidual in the emotional and psychological space which is currently hers. This does seem a sensible place to be as a midwife, becoming an ally and advocate for the woman and her unborn child, rather than taking a particular viewpoint on the best route to take medically.

The case also highlights the dangers associated with making assumptions about what a patient would want, based on our own experiences and preferences. While it can be helpful to imagine what a patient may be feeling, there is no way of understanding what they are thinking and what their choice of action might be until all potential interventions are discussed and the risks and benefits of all options are weighed up. Until this point, the patient cannot make a fully informed choice. Ultimately, it is the patient and their family who will have to live with the consequences of whatever choices are made, and therefore, it is essential that we support the decision-making process in an open-minded way, regardless of our personal preferences, choices, and beliefs. Parents need clear, unbiased information about their choices and the options available to them. Women and their partners may feel psychologically and emotionally overwhelmed (Roberts et al., 2007). Both pregnancy and a cancer diagnosis are life-changing events; while the physical well-being of the woman is a high priority, the psychological aspect of her care is vitally important (Howe et al., 2022).

Although rare, cancer in pregnancy has been increasing in recent years (Botha et al. 2018). Cervical cancer is the most commonly occurring cancer encountered during pregnancy, with an estimated incidence of 0.8–1.5 cases per 10,000 births (Singh et al., 2023). This may be because women are delaying childbearing (Tang et al., 2024). The condition requires a multidisciplinary approach (Le Guévelou et al., 2024).

The management of cervical cancer during pregnancy is very challenging because of the physiological changes that take place during pregnancy (Amant et al., 2019). Symptoms may therefore be masked due to hormonal changes. It is therefore imperative that pregnant women remain vigilant to vaginal bleeding in pregnancy and to any abnormal vaginal discharge. It is also challenging because of the dual stakes of treating the cancer without compromising the health of the foetus (Le Guévelou et al., 2024). Diagnosis is usually made in the second trimester (Ma et al., 2019). In a systematic review, Dąbrowska et al. (2024) found that many women chose termination of pregnancy, some chose combination therapy, some chose chemotherapy, very few patients chose radiotherapy, and one patient refused treatment. The type of treatment is going to depend on the gestational age, disease stage, and the patient's personal preference (Han et al., 2013).

In the recent confidential enquiry into maternal death (Felker et al., 2024), three women died from cervical cancer in the period 2020–2022. The authors suggest that women diagnosed with cancer during pregnancy should be investigated in the same manner as a non-pregnant woman. The National Institute for Health and Care Excellence (NICE, 2023) states that a woman should be referred for an appointment within two weeks if cervical cancer is suspected. The confidential enquiry team also suggests that when women experience vaginal bleeding in pregnancy, a cause coincidental to the pregnancy should be considered, and most imaging and treatments for cancer are safe during pregnancy and should not be delayed (Felker et al., 2024). The Royal College of Obstetricians and Gynaecologists (RCOG) recommends that if a woman presents with a clinically suspicious cervix, she should be referred for colposcopic evaluation (RCOG green top guideline 63, 2011).

There is no "blueprint" for the right thing to do. Each woman is an individual and considered carefully on this basis.

Questions for reflection and discussion

Explore the key issues raised in the above scenario as you answer the following six questions:

1. How would you find the balance between enabling shared decision-making and avoiding giving false hope, which may arise in situations like Erica's?

2. To what extent do you think people diagnosed with cancer who are having to make difficult decisions are guided by a mixture of feelings, beliefs, and personal values, as opposed to the objective weighing up of risks?

3. In terms of forming a therapeutic relationship with Erica and patients in a similar situation, what are the risks associated with making assumptions about the approach she wants to take or persuading her to take what we consider the most rational approach?

4. What does this case tell us about the importance of patients being fully informed about the risks and benefits of possible interventions and approaches to treatment within pregnancy?

5. What are the benefits and challenges of working with patients who have a high level of digital health literacy?

6. Consider what you know about cancer in pregnancy and whether you feel you would require further training to manage this situation.

Further reading

Huang, H., Quan, Y., Qi, X. and Liu, P. (2021) Neoadjuvant chemotherapy with paclitaxel plus cisplatin before radical surgery for locally advanced cervical cancer during pregnancy: A case series and literature review. *Medicine* 100(*32*): e26845, DOI: 10.1097/MD.0000000000026845

Macdonald S. and Johnson G. (eds) (2017) *Mayes' Midwifery* (15th Edition) Elsevier.

Marshall J. and Raynor M. (eds) (2020) *Myles Textbook for Midwives* (17th Edition) Elsevier.

Robson S. and Waugh J. (eds) (2013) *Medical Disorders in Pregnancy: A Manual for Midwives.* Wiley Blackwell.

Rodrigo, S.G., Calderon, J., Dionisi, J.N., Santi, A., Mariconde, J.M., Rosato, O.D. and Amant, F. (2021) Cervical cancer in pregnancy at various gestational ages. *International Journal of Gynecological Cancer*, 31(*5*): 784–788.

Further information

VALUES

Care involves practitioners engaging in interactions and interventions which focus on the needs of the person within their context. Caring also includes making use of an evidence-based approach to providing the right care, in a timely way, at every stage of life.

Compassion is defined in Compassion in Practice as "how care is given through relationships based on empathy, respect and dignity" (Department of Health, 2012, p. 13).

Consent should be asked for in all circumstances, with appropriate and full information being provided in order to enable an informed choice.

Curiosity involves going beyond what is immediately obvious by observing, listening, asking questions, and reflecting on the information gathered.

Hope has been described as an integral part of being human and is seen as having three main dimensions: firstly, an inner power that enables people to transcend their present situation; secondly, the anticipation of an improved state; and lastly, as a personal experience, centred on our chances of achieving what we want (Antunes et al., 2023).

Respect involves recognising and acknowledging the unconditional value of all people living with cancer as persons in a way which enables them to maintain their dignity and self-respect.

THEORIES

Digital health literacy involves being able to find, understand, and make use of health information from sources such as the Internet, allowing patients to make more informed decisions about their health or to manage their conditions more effectively.

Emotional labour in healthcare is a term which recognises the work healthcare professionals put into managing their own emotions to present as calm and caring to patients, even when needing to suppress their own feelings, by prioritising the emotional needs of their patients.

Emotional support recognises that expressing emotions and the feelings involved in living with a cancer diagnosis, including coping with circumstances which sometimes change rapidly, are fundamental aspects of providing person-centred care.

Social norms arise from the beliefs, attitudes, and behaviours considered acceptable in a particular social group or culture and which provide guidelines on how to behave in a range of social situations, therefore leading to greater order and a certain amount of predictability in society and social relationships. Most people experience considerable social pressure to conform to the prevailing norms in any given situation.

Social stigma refers to something being seen as a social disgrace, as outlined by Erving Goffman (1963). Goffman considered that stigma is an attribute that extensively discredits an individual, reducing him or her from someone seen as a whole person to someone seen as being tainted, who is discounted for the label that makes them stand out from others.

APPROACHES

Active listening is an essential aspect of respecting patients. Becoming an effective listener involves actively engaging with people to make sense of what we see in their body language, in combination with what we hear. We need to hear, consider, and process what is said to us in nursing, and this is never a passive process (Ali, 2018).

Avoid making assumptions: Stenhouse (2021, p. 27) states that practitioners "must treat people as individuals, avoid making assumptions about them, recognise diversity and individual choice, and respect and uphold their dignity and human rights."

Empathy is essential for providing person-centred care. It enables the person providing support to better understand the world from the perspective of the patient and, therefore, to respond to their experience of service delivery with an individualised approach.

Human rights are outlined by the British Institute of Human Rights (2014), which advocates using a human rights-based approach to working with people living with cancer, including implementation of the PANEL framework:

- *Participation* – everyone has the right to participate actively and meaningfully in decisions which affect them. Participation must give attention to issues of accessibility, including access to information in a form and a language which can be understood.

- *Accountability* – the need for effective monitoring of human rights standards as well as effective remedies for human rights breaches.

- *Non-discrimination and equality* – all discrimination in the realisation of rights must be prohibited, prevented, and eliminated.

- *Empowerment* – individuals and communities should understand their rights and should be fully supported to participate in the development of policies and practices which affect their lives.

- *Legality* – rights are recognised as legally enforceable and are linked to national and international human rights law.

Lifespan approach recognises the temporal dimension of health, rather than just distinct episodes of illness, personalising and humanising health scenarios as part of a life process. It emphasises health promotion, ill-health prevention and well-being, as well as management of ill-health throughout life.

Patient-centred goal planning takes a collaborative approach, with documentation showing how people and their representatives of choice are supported to be involved in developing and reviewing progress towards establishing and meeting personally meaningful goals.

Recognising feelings through sympathetic awareness of another person's experiences is central to providing person-centred care, as well as to providing approaches which help to avoid unnecessary stress or distress in people who have received a cancer diagnosis.

Shared decision-making focuses on including patients in all decisions about their own lives so that their voices are heard and their individual preferences understood and fully represented in any decision-making process which takes place.

Teamwork involves more than working alongside health practitioners from other professions or at a different stage of their careers. It also provides opportunities for taking into consideration different professional perspectives of relevance to decision-making and reflection on and in practice to improve patient outcomes.

Validation recognises the importance of validating the emotional aspects and expressed feelings within the experiences of people. Thus, while a practitioner may not agree with a patient about an aspect of their care, it is nonetheless helpful to connect with the feelings which the person has about the situation.

MODELS

Non-verbal communication includes gestures, facial expressions, movements, muscle tension, and posture, alongside the volume, tone, and pitch of vocalisations. Each person has an individual profile of non-verbal communication, although there may be some culturally and socially derived gestures and expressions which people from similar backgrounds share.

Person-centred practice is an approach to working with people which provides dignity, respect, and choice.

Stages of cervical cancer as defined by the International Federation of Gynaecology and Obstetrics (FIGO) are:

Stage I (2018): Carcinoma strictly confined to the cervix.

Stage II (2018): Carcinoma invades beyond the uterus but has not extended onto the lower third of the vagina or to the pelvic wall.

Stage III (2018): Carcinoma involves the lower third of the vagina and/or extends to the pelvic wall and/or causes hydronephrosis or non-functioning kidney and/or involves pelvic and/or para-aortic lymph nodes.

Stage IV (2018): Carcinoma has extended beyond the true pelvis or has involved (biopsy-proven) the mucosa of the bladder or rectum.

References

Ali, M. (2018). Communication Skills 5: Effective listening and observation. *Nursing Times* [online]. 114(*4*): 56–57.

Amant, F., Berveiller, P., Boere, I. A., Cardonick, E., Fruscio, R., Fumagalli, M., and Zapardiel, I. (2019). Gynecologic cancers in pregnancy: Guidelines based on a third international consensus meeting. *Annals of Oncology*. 30(*10*): 1601–1612.

Antunes, M., Laranjeira, C., Querido, A. and Charepe, Z. (2023). "What do we know about hope in nursing care?": A synthesis of concept analysis studies. *Healthcare* (Basel). 11(*20*): 2739. doi: 10.3390/healthcare11202739. PMID: 37893813; PMCID: PMC10606526.

Botha, M.H., Rajaram, S. and Karunaratne, K. (2018). Cancer in pregnancy. *International Journal of Gynecology & Obstetrics*. 143: 137–142.

British Institute of Human Rights (2014). *The Difference It Makes: Putting Human Rights at the Heart of Health and Social Care*. Available at: https://www.bihr.org.uk/media/4w3bqxcj/putting_human_rights_at_heart_of_health_and_care.pdf (Accessed 30th June 2025).

Dąbrowska, A., Perdyan, A., Sobocki, B.K. and Rutkowski, J. (2024). Management of cervical cancer during pregnancy – A systematic review. *Biuletyn Polskiego Towarzystwa Onkologicznego Nowotwory*. 9(*1*): 27–33.

Department of Health (2012). *Compassion in Practice: Nursing, Midwifery and Care Staff: Our Vision and Strategy*. London: Gateway reference 18479.

Felker, A., Patel, R., Kotnis, R., Kenyon, S. and Knight, M. (Eds.) on behalf of MBRRACE-UK. *Saving Lives, Improving Mothers' Care Compiled Report – Lessons Learned to Inform Maternity Care from the UK and Ireland Confidential Enquiries into Maternal Deaths and Morbidity* 2020–22. Oxford: National Perinatal Epidemiology Unit, University of Oxford 2024.

Goffman, E. (1963/1990). *Stigma: Notes on the Management of Spoiled Identity*. London: Penguin.

Han, S.N., Mhallem Gziri, M., Van Calsteren, K. and Amant, F. (2013). Cervical cancer in pregnant women: Treat, wait or interrupt? Assessment of current clinical guidelines, innovations and controversies. *Therapeutic Advances in Medical Oncology*. 5(*4*): 211–219.

Howe, T., Lankester, K., Kelly, T., Watkins, R. and Kaushik, S. (2022). Cervical cancer in pregnancy: diagnosis, staging and treatment. *The Obstetrician & Gynaecologist*. 24(*1*), 31–39.

Le Guévelou, J., Selleret, L., Laas, E., Lecuru, F. and Kissel, M. (2024). Cervical cancer associated with pregnancy: Current challenges and future strategies. *Cancers*. 16(*7*): 1341.

Ma, J., Yu, L., Xu, F., Yi, H., Wei, W., Wu, P. and Fan, L. (2019). Treatment and clinical outcomes of cervical cancer during pregnancy. *Annals of Translational Medicine*. 7(*11*): 241

National Institute for Health and Clinical Excellence Suspected Cancer Recognition and Referral (2023). www.nice.org.uk/guidance/ng12

Roberts, K., Rezai, N. and Edmondson, R.J. (2007). Cervical cancer in pregnancy: An assault on family and fertility. *British Journal of Midwifery*. 15(*3*): 132–136.

Royal College of Obstetricians and Gynaecologists (RCOG) (2011). Antepartum Haemorrhage (Green-top Guideline No. 63).

Singh, D., Vignat, J., Lorenzoni, V., Eslahi, M., Ginsburg, O., Lauby-Secretan, B. and Vaccarella, S. (2023). Global estimates of incidence and mortality of cervical cancer in 2020: A baseline analysis of the WHO Global Cervical Cancer Elimination Initiative. *The Lancet Global Health*. 11(2): e197–e206.

Stenhouse, R. (2021). Understanding equality and diversity in nursing practice. *Nursing Standard* (Royal College of Nursing, Great Britain). 36(*2*), 27–33. https://doi.org/10.7748/ns.2020.e11562

Tang, X., Zhang, X., Ding, Y., Zhang, Y., Zhang, N., Qiu, J. and Hua, K. (2024). A long-term retrospective analysis of management of cervical cancer during pregnancy. *International Journal of Gynecology & Obstetrics*. 165(*3*): 1189–1198.

Case study 7
Michelle: adjusting to bodily change

Jennie Burch and Gabrielle Thorpe

Another day, another clinic

I read the referral letter about Michelle, who has an appointment to see me, the clinical nurse specialist (CNS) in stoma
care, in the preoperative stoma care clinic today. It had
been a busy morning, and I still feel residual stress from
a difficult encounter earlier. I try to calm myself with several deep breaths to focus on Michelle. Michelle is 45 years
of age and scheduled to undergo a low anterior resection
for a low rectal cancer. This means that she will need her
rectum and part of her sigmoid colon removed. The colorectal surgeon will then anastomose (join) the bowel to the
small amount of remaining distal rectum. The magnetic
resonance imaging (MRI) scan shows the cancer to be
stage 3. This means that the cancer is locally advanced,
having spread to the nearby lymph nodes, so Michelle will
need chemotherapy as well as surgery.

VALUE: professionalism

VALUE: self-awareness

In the referral letter, I would expect to read definitively that
Michelle needs a temporary ileostomy, as in my Trust, it is
common practice when operating on a low rectal cancer
to form a temporary ileostomy. Instead, the referral letter
reads that Michelle might need a temporary stoma. I sigh
inwardly; this is not setting Michelle's expectations very
well for my consultation. The clinic appointment is planned
to be an hour. The aim of the clinic appointment is to provide information and preoperative stoma bag management
training. Surgery is planned for next week.

APPROACH: informed consent

VALUE: accountability

Welcoming Michelle

I open the clinic room door and walk to where I assume
Michelle is sitting. A middle-aged woman is alone in the
waiting room, and I ask if she is Michelle. A pair of scared
eyes looks at me, and she nods her head. 'Please come
in,' I direct her brightly. Michelle's demeanour is one of

DOI: 10.4324/9781003651758-7

sadness, and I think to myself that one hour will not be sufficient today.

APPROACH: therapeutic relationship

I introduce myself and my role to Michelle. I have barely finished when Michelle interjects, saying, 'Stoma nurse? The doctor told me there was a good chance that I won't need one. I don't want one! I would rather die!' Michelle sounds hopeless, and I am not expecting her to say this, but I want to know more about why she feels this way. Michelle states in a shrill voice, 'A stoma is disgusting! I will smell! I am too young to have a stoma!' I let Michelle continue speaking about her fears of surgery and having a stoma without interruption, nodding so that she will know she is heard, until she comes to a natural end. I summarise Michelle's concerns back to her, beginning by saying, 'What I am hearing is ....' to ensure I have understood her. I conclude after this summary: 'This is such a challenging position to be in, no wonder you feel a bit overwhelmed.' Michelle nods and looks down.

THEORY: hopelessness

THEORY: emotional intelligence

THEORY: uncertainty

APPROACH: sensitivity

APPROACH: active listening

APPROACH: non-judgemental

APPROACH: active listening

APPROACH: affirming

MODEL: SPIKES

APPROACH: empathy

APPROACH: informed consent

VALUE: professionalism

THEORY: unconscious bias

I choose the SPIKES model to discuss Michelle's bad news, which I find particularly useful when I am having discussions with distressed patients. I gently ask Michelle if I can explain about what would happen to her and why things might be necessary during her rectal cancer treatment pathway. She nods again, but this time Michelle keeps her head up. I consider it important that Michelle has all the information needed to make an informed decision about her cancer treatment. Michelle does not fit my preconception of someone who wants to refuse treatment, and I am sure she has the capacity to make decisions. My assumption is based on the fact that Michelle had previously noted a change in bowel habit and experienced an episode of rectal bleeding, and these symptoms prompted her to visit her general practitioner (GP). Michelle's GP recognised potential signs of colorectal cancer and referred her on a cancer pathway to the hospital for investigations. I consider, therefore, that Michelle does not fit the profile of a person who might choose not to have cancer treatment, as this group includes people with comorbidities, limited education, a low income, and people of increasing age. Michelle is not part of this group.

APPROACH: evidence-based practice

I wonder whether Michelle has not heard or retained all the information explained to her by the doctor in the surgical clinic, or maybe the doctor has not given her sufficient information for her needs. It is important to provide pre-operative information to reduce anxiety and increase preparedness for surgery. Education and counselling before colorectal surgery are important for patients, although it can be difficult to understand information in emotional situations when the patient is feeling shocked at their cancer diagnosis. As about half of people diagnosed with cancer show significant levels of distress, it is a usual part of my role to speak to people who need more information about their colorectal cancer journey.

VALUE: communication

APPROACH: informed consent

APPROACH: empathy

Exploring Michelle's understanding

To establish what Michelle already knows about her cancer diagnosis, I ask her to explain what the doctor has already told her. Michelle seems to become more distant as she speaks. Thinking about the Kubler-Ross stages of grief, I recognise that Michelle might be in the denial and isolation phase. Although this stage of grief, when it occurs, can help people cope with their circumstances and maintain hope of recovery, I am concerned that it might prevent Michelle from being able to take in new information during this consultation. Michelle's explanation shows that she has a reasonable understanding of her cancer and the need for treatment but does not understand the specific treatment proposed nor the potential consequences of the interventions. I am also able to establish that Michelle understands reasonably complex explanations, which I hope will continue during our consultation.

THEORY: grief

VALUE: compassion

VALUE: respect

I need to explain the cancer treatment plan in a way that will enable Michelle to understand and make an informed decision about treatment. My hope is that she will accept the treatment option that will give her the best chance of long-term survival, which will almost certainly include the formation of a temporary ileostomy. I need to communicate to her in a manner that enables Michelle to not just understand but also to make the necessary psychological adjustments to determine the cancer treatment choices

VALUE: honesty

that she is able to accept. Taking a deep breath, I begin my explanation of Michelle's treatment plan.

I begin my explanation with slight nervousness, as I am uncertain how Michelle will react to my direct approach: 'Michelle, I have heard how you feel about having a stoma, and I understand your concerns. But I would really like to help you to understand in more detail what your cancer treatment plan will look like. Can I start with exploring bowel anatomy?' I take out a piece of paper and begin to draw the colon, rectum, and anus, adding a shaded area in the lower rectum to indicate the position of the cancer. Visual aids often improve a patient's understanding of their anatomy and the need for surgery.

APPROACH: validation

VALUE: communication

Michelle points at the image and asks, 'Is this where my cancer is?' which shows she has understood the drawing. I confirm this and explain the way in which the colon and rectum work, how poo is moved towards the anus and what it means to have her rectum removed. Michelle was listening, and when I checked for her understanding, she had no additional questions at this time.

VALUE: honesty

VALUE: communication

Next, I want to explore the cancer treatment and how it will affect her bowel function. This will include discussing the risks and benefits of having the rectal resection. I am more anxious about this part of the discussion because it involves discussing the stoma, but I feel we are beginning to develop a therapeutic relationship. In my experience, it is more likely for patients to comprehend the need for the stoma once we develop some trust between us. I want to be direct about the aims of cancer treatment and try and make this sound positive. I begin hesitantly, 'So Michelle, the aim of having cancer treatment is to remove all the visible cancer and then probably to have more treatment, possibly chemotherapy, to remove all the tiny cancer cells that we cannot see.' I check this is her understanding and, more importantly, her desire for her treatment goal, which she confirms.

APPROACH: therapeutic relationship

VALUE: trust

I continue to explain in more detail about the surgery, and I am happy that Michelle seems to be coping well with my direct approach to information provision. I need to explore the risks and benefits of the operation, and this is where I usually add information about the stoma. I explain, 'Michelle, we have talked about the benefits of treatment; I am now going to explain some of the risks of having the cancer removed during the low anterior resection. You can see how close your cancer is to your anal canal.' I say, pointing at my diagram, then continue, 'All of this is within your pelvic bones. This makes it difficult for the surgeon to reach. What that means is even for a good surgeon, which yours is, about one in every ten people will have a problem with the join in the bowel, such as a leak. Having a leak is obviously not a good thing, as it means poo can leave your bowel and go inside of you. This can make you very poor, and if this happens, it is common to need another operation. This is why the surgeon will probably, in my experience, choose to divert the flow of the bowel and form a temporary stoma to make sure you don't get very poorly if a problem does happen.' I stop to ensure that I still have Michelle's attention and that she is still listening. She seems more receptive now to the thought of having a stoma than at the beginning of the consultation. I have been directed, but I hope that this approach is acceptable to Michelle. It seems to be. I, therefore, explain about the stoma, adopting the same matter-of-fact approach that seems to have worked so far.

APPROACH: informed consent

APPROACH: evidence-based practice

VALUE: honesty

Michelle has a lot of questions, which I answer one by one. I can feel she is beginning to accept the idea of having a stoma. I am relieved, as it will be in her best interest to have a temporary stoma, particularly as she will need chemotherapy, and any postoperative complication could delay or prevent this adjuvant therapy.

APPROACH: empowerment

THEORY: psychological adjustment

I check in with Michelle, asking what it is about the stoma that concerns her the most. Odour is one issue, so this feels like the right time to show her an ileostomy bag to reduce this concern. Being made from plastic, stoma bags are secure and very different from stoma bags of the past. Michelle takes the bag and handles it. It seems to me that this helps her. She is not scared to touch the bag. I ask Michelle what she thinks of the bag. Michelle replies in an

APPROACH: person-centred care

almost relieved manner: 'Well, it is smaller and lighter than I expected. This is not what I expected, I am not quite sure what I did expect, but not this.' It feels right to continue.

APPROACH: active listening

When I explain to Michelle how the ileostomy bag will stick on her tummy to collect the poo, she becomes quiet again before saying, 'I am going to look terrible with a bag of poo stuck on me.' Body image can be an issue for people with a stoma, not simply the stoma bag but also the abdominal scars. It is important for healthcare professionals to assist people with a stoma to adapt and achieve an acceptable quality of life, which can be difficult when there are issues with their body image. In addition to living with an altered body image, there can be issues relating to the lack of control of bowel function and alterations in the embodied self with discord between how people see a unity between their body, themselves, and the world. I reassure Michelle that these feelings are common for many people planning to have a stoma formation. To reduce these negative feelings and facilitate adaptation, people learn to adjust to having a stoma by taking control, such as through mastering the stoma bag change technique. It is important for the nurse to recognise and facilitate adaptation to life with the stoma to minimise these negative feelings and promote self-acceptance.

THEORY: body image

THEORY: embodied self

APPROACH: validation

THEORY: self-determination

VALUE: acceptance

I explained to Michelle that the ileostomy bag would be emptied regularly and it should not be visible under clothing. This seems to reduce her concerns somewhat. I think this is the right time to suggest pulling a stoma appliance on Michelle's abdomen. I hope she is agreeable. 'Michelle', I say, 'would it be helpful to try putting on an ileostomy bag and see how you feel once it is stuck on your tummy?' Michelle seems uncertain but is willing to try. I reach across the desk for the stoma pack, which contains a fake stoma made from foam stuck on an adhesive base as well as an ileostomy bag. Michelle follows my instruction and sticks the foam stoma onto her abdomen in the place where the ileostomy would be. Michelle then successfully measures the fake stoma and carefully places an ileostomy bag over her 'stoma' and zips up her trousers. There is a visible reduction in tension between my initial suggestion

APPROACH: goal setting

THEORY: self-determination

of Michelle putting the ileostomy bag onto her abdomen and now. I ask Michelle how she feels now she has the ileostomy bag on. She replies, 'I can't say I like it, but it does not feel as bulky and scary as I expected.'

Setting expectations

My last activity for this preoperative session is to set expectations appropriately on two further points. Firstly, Michelle will need to be self-caring for her stoma appliance, and secondly, to provide her with information about her likely bowel function after the stoma is reversed. For the first point, I hope Michelle is feeling more confident after applying the fake stoma and that she will assume that she will be expected to self-manage her ileostomy at home. When I ask her, Michelle says: 'I think I can master this stoma bag; I am quite determined.' This was a great starting point. I am also concerned about the level of support available to Michelle away from the hospital, as I know supportive friends and family can help people adjust better to their stoma. To determine this, I ask her, 'Who can offer you support at home?' to which she replies that she has good support from her family and friends. This pleases and reassures me, as it seems that Michelle is beginning to accept the thought of having a stoma and that she has the support needed to adapt successfully to living with a stoma. I give Michelle a leaflet to remind her about the points we have discussed.

THEORY: self-determination

MODEL: motivational interviewing

THEORY: coping

I explain that I also need to give Michelle some information about common changes to bowel function after having treatment for her rectal cancer. I know it is important to set expectations correctly and ensure that people understand that their bowel function is likely to change after most of the rectum is removed. This enables them to make choices before an operation that could include choosing to have a permanent stoma, because for that individual the thought of bowel dysfunction may be more troublesome than having a colostomy. I do not think that Michelle will choose this option, but I think she needs to have the information to enable her to make an informed choice about her rectal cancer treatment options.

APPROACH: empowerment

APPROACH: informed consent

I explain that because of the changes in anatomy created by the removal of the rectum, there would also be a change in function, as there would be less storage for the poo. There might also be changes in how the nerves work because of the surgery and other treatments she might need, such as chemotherapy. I describe how her bowel function might alter, explaining that she will be likely to poo more often and that her bowel function will be less predictable, certainly in the short term. In addition, I add that things will improve with time and that there are lots of ways to help improve bowel function when the changes do occur. Again, I want to enable her to be informed, independent, and self-caring with the consequences of cancer treatment, as I know all these points will help her to have an improved quality of life.

I ask Michelle to summarise what she expects her bowel function to be after the stoma is reversed, and she states, 'I think there may be some problems, but I think I can handle them. Will I have someone to help me if I need it?' I confirm that the cancer nurse will be there for advice from now until three years after her surgery, and I will be there to help with any stoma issues, as well as the surgeon and oncologist.

The last thing I needed was to make plans for Michelle. We need to determine if she would like another opportunity to discuss her stoma in the clinic or whether she would just like to have the site of the stoma marked and an opportunity for any last questions on the day of admission. Michelle thinks she is okay and can leave it to her admission day. I say, 'That is a great plan, Michelle.' She smiles for the first time since I met her.

Reflections

After the session with Michelle, I reflected on how commonly distress is experienced by people facing treatment for cancer. This is often considered to be part of the five stages of grief described by Kubler-Ross (Tyrrell et al., 2023). While I did not think that Michelle had come through to the final acceptance phase, I did feel that she had heard what I had to say and left with more knowledge and fewer concerns than she had when she entered the clinic room. I also reflected on my inability to accurately assess Michelle in terms of grief and distress. I had not used a validated tool to detect distress as described by Simnacher et al. (2023). I was simply working on my experience and was not certain if this was enough evidence on which to base my decisions. This is something I should consider when I see people after discharge home with their stoma, as some people cope better than others, and it is known that the first three to six months after surgery can be a difficult time.

I also reflected on how I can improve my communication skills within clinical practice. Motivational interviewing is a skill that I think will be helpful to use more to assist patients on the journey towards independent self-care (Miller and Rollnick, 2023). Some of those skills I already use in clinical practice, such as active listening and the use of open-ended questions, but I also need to consider other skills, such as helping patients to explore and become motivated to change.

Questions for reflection and discussion

Explore the key issues raised in the above scenario as you answer the following six questions:

1. Reflect on the range of concerns people planning to have a stoma formation might have.

2. Discuss the stages of grief, how they apply to different aspects of cancer treatment and care, and why they might vary for individuals.

3. Reflect on ways you can support and facilitate an improvement in body image for a person living with a stoma.

4. Discuss how your clinical environment might better support people experiencing emotional distress or a low mood after a cancer diagnosis.

5. In what ways could the individual, their family and friends, and the healthcare team help to improve quality of life for a person living with a stoma?

6. Discuss ways of enabling patients in the ward environment to have better access to toilets after rectal cancer surgery.

Further reading

Alenezi, A., McGrath, I., Kimpton, A. and Livesay, K. (2021) Quality of life among ostomy patients: A narrative literature review. *Journal of Clinical Nursing*, 30(21–22): 3111–3123.

Burch, J., Bird, A. and Thorpe, G. (2024) The role of the clinical nurse specialist in stoma care: A modified Delphi consensus. *Journal of Advanced Nursing*, 80(8): 3371–3381. https://doi:10.1111/jan.16032.

Mathew, A., Doorenbos, A.Z. and Vincent, C. (2021) Symptom management theory: Analysis, evaluation, and implications for caring for adults with cancer. *ANS Advanced Nursing Science*, 44(3): E93–E112. https://doi:10.1097/ANS.0000000000000347.

Petersén, C. and Carlsson, E. (2021) Life with a stoma-coping with daily life: Experiences from focus group interviews. *Journal of Clinical Nursing*, 30(15–16): 2309–2319.

Thorpe, G., Arthur, A. and McArthur, M. (2016) Adjusting to bodily change following stoma formation: A phenomenological study. *Disability & Rehabilitation*, 38(18): 1791–1802.

Further information

VALUES

Acceptance is central to person-centred practice. It sits alongside being non-judgemental and understanding the perspective of the person as a central tenet of working with people living with cancer as they present throughout their illness trajectories. It is key to promoting patient well-being.

Accountability is the act of being responsible for personal actions.

Autonomy is a fundamental principle in medical ethics, granting individuals the right to make decisions about their healthcare without undue influence from providers. It encompasses informed consent, which requires patients to voluntarily agree to treatment after receiving comprehensive information.

Communication is 'central to successful caring relationships and to effective team working. Listening is as important as what we say and do' (Department of Health, 2012, p. 13).

Compassion is defined in Compassion in Practice as 'how care is given through relationships based on empathy, respect and dignity' (Department of Health, 2012, p. 13).

Honesty is an essential quality in any person working in healthcare due to the vulnerability of service users, many of whom will be living with long-term illnesses or conditions, which may make them fully or partially dependent on the care and support of others.

Professionalism leads to 'the consistent provision of safe, effective, person-centred outcomes that support people and their families and carers to achieve an optimal status of health and well-being' (NMC, 2016, p. 3).

Respect involves recognising and acknowledging the unconditional value of all people in a way which enables them to maintain their dignity and self-respect.

Self-awareness of practitioners providing health and care services is integral to reflective practice, delivering person-centred care, and the therapeutic use of self to build relationships focused on a shared understanding of things which are important to the patient.

Teamworking is a vital aspect of cancer care, ensuring that comprehensive and coordinated care is delivered to meet the complex needs of each individual. Effective communication is essential within teamwork, as nurses need to share information accurately and in a timely manner to ensure seamless care.

Trust is reliance on character, including the belief that somebody is good and honest.

THEORIES

Body image can be defined as a person's internal picture of what their own body looks like. For some people, this will be closely connected to their social confidence, sense of self-esteem, and self-identity.

Embodied self is a sense of self based on the integral and unconscious unity of body and mind. When the integrity of the body is limited or challenged through disease or disability, it can be perceived to be encumbered and constrained. This forces the body to be experienced consciously and can limit the capacity of the self to operate within the freedoms it previously experienced.

Emotional intelligence (EI) is the ability to recognise, understand, and manage emotions in oneself and others. It encompasses skills such as identifying and discriminating among emotions and using emotional information to guide thinking and actions. Some researchers suggest that EI can be learned and strengthened, while others argue it is an innate characteristic.

Hope has been described as an integral part of being human and is seen as having three main dimensions: firstly, an inner power that enables people to transcend their present situation; secondly, the anticipation of an improved state; and lastly, as a personal experience centred on our chances of achieving what we want (Antunes et al., 2023).

Psychological adjustment relates to a person's acceptance of changes in their physical, occupational, and/or social environment, which may include adjustment of self-perception, modifying personal beliefs and goals, and compensating for any residual disability by developing appropriate strategies.

Self-determination theory is a theory of motivation introduced by Deci and Ryan (1985) based on three essential needs of competence, autonomy, and relatedness.

Uncertainty – Uncertainty Management Theory is a communication theory by Brashers (2001) which focuses on three components: the experience and meaning of uncertainty, appraisal of and emotional responses to uncertainty, and behavioural adaptation to uncertainty.

Unconscious bias is a form of social stereotyping about certain groups of people, formed outside of conscious awareness. Due to the tendency of humans to organise the social world by categorising people into groups, everyone holds unconscious beliefs about the various social and identity groups they come across.

APPROACHES

Active listening involves not simply listening but showing you are interested in listening by making eye contact, not interrupting, and not being judgemental, as well as asking questions.

Affirming is to declare support for something or make an emphatic statement about something. Often used in healthcare as part of a communication approach to encourage a person to feel confident about making their own decisions.

Care planning is a systematic approach to care involving the comprehensive assessment of a person's care needs, identification of defined care goals, a plan of actions and interventions that will meet defined goals of care, and evaluating the extent to which goals have been met.

Empathy is essential for providing person-centred care. It enables the person providing support to better understand the world from the perspective of the patient and, therefore, to respond to their experience of service delivery with an individualised approach.

Empowerment is a concept that promotes autonomous self-regulation and maximises an individual's potential for health and wellness. It involves patients gaining knowledge, skills, and attitudes to actively participate in their healthcare decisions and improve their quality of life.

Goal setting is the process used to identify specific and measurable objectives.

Hopelessness is a feeling or state of despair. Hopelessness, by definition, is the belief that things are not going to get better or that you cannot succeed.

Informed consent is a critical component in providing patient-centred care in healthcare settings. These processes ensure that patients are fully informed and agree to the care or procedures being performed.

Non-judgemental care acknowledges individuality and holism and all aspects of people's lives. The values involved in non-judgemental care are acceptance, empathy, and sincerity. Acceptance is about respecting the person's feelings, experiences, and values, even though they may differ from yours. The Nursing and Midwifery Council (2018) stresses that nurses must practise in a holistic, non-judgemental, caring, and sensitive manner that avoids assumptions and supports social inclusion, recognises and respects individual choice, and acknowledges diversity.

Patient-centred care is an approach focusing on the whole person, including factors such as their emotions, preferences, values, and sociocultural circumstances, alongside their immediate symptoms and health needs.

Sensitivity is an important approach to maintain in healthcare since being sensitive in communication is being considerate about what is said and how it is said and being receptive to how the other person is engaging with you in the conversation. This allows you the opportunity to refine your message and its delivery.

Therapeutic relationship describes the relationship between a healthcare professional and a person for whom they are caring, in which the focus of the relationship is on the person receiving care.

Validation can be used by a healthcare professional to communicate with a person receiving care to check that they have accurately interpreted a person's thoughts, feelings, beliefs, and preferences.

MODELS

Motivational interviewing – a counselling technique developed by psychologists Miller and Rollnick (1991) to encourage a person to make positive changes to their behaviour by exploring factors contributing to the person's ambivalence about behaviour change and directing them to consider how they might achieve their goals.

SPIKES is an acronym to guide an organised discussion when delivering distressing information (bad news) to patients. The SPIKES model (Mills et al., 2024) reminds the healthcare professional to consider the clinical **S**etting, the patient's **P**erception, to **I**nvite questions, provide **K**nowledge, validate **E**motions, and **S**ummarise discussions.

References

Antunes, M., Laranjeira, C., Querido, A. and Charepe, Z. (2023) "What Do We Know about Hope in Nursing Care?": A Synthesis of Concept Analysis Studies. *Healthcare (Basel)*, 11(20): 2739. doi: 10.3390/healthcare11202739. PMID: 37893813; PMCID: PMC10606526.

Brashers, D. (2001) Communication and Uncertainty Management. *Journal of Communication*, 51(3): 477–497. doi: 10.1111/j.1460-2466.2001.tb02892.x

Deci, E.L. and Ryan, R.M. (1985) *Intrinsic Motivation and Self-Determination in Human Behavior*. New York: Springer.

Department of Health (2012) *Compassion in Practice; Nursing, Midwifery and Care Staff; Our Vision and Strategy*. London: Gateway reference 18479.

Miller, W.R. and Rollnick, S. (1991) *Motivational Interviewing: Preparing People to Change Addictive Behavior*. New York: Guilford Press.

Mills, L.M., Cate, O.T., Boscardin, C. and O'Sullivan, P.S. (2024) Breaking Bad News to Learners: How Well Does the SPIKES Clinical Model Translate? *Perspect Medical Education*, 13(1): 684–692. doi: 10.5334/pme.1521.

NMC (2016) Enabling Professionalism in Nursing and Midwifery Practice, Available at: https://www.nmc.org.uk/globalassets/sitedocuments/other-publications/enabling-professionalism.pdf (Accessed 19th February 2024).

Nursing and Midwifery Council (NMC) (2018) The Code: Professional Standards of Practice and Behaviour for Nurses, Midwives and Nursing Associates. Available at: https://www.nmc.org.uk (Accessed 30th June 2025).

Simnacher, F., Götz, A., Kling, S., Schulze, J.B., von Känel, R., Euler, S. and Günther, M.P. (2023) A Short Screening Tool Identifying Systemic Barriers to Distress Screening in Cancer Care. *Cancer Medicine*, 12(16): 17313–17321.

Tyrrell, P., Harberger, S., Schoo, C. and Siddiqui, W. (2023) *Kubler-Ross Stages of Dying and Subsequent Models of Grief*. StatPearls. Available at: https://www.ncbi.nlm.nih.gov/books/NBK+85/

Case study 8
Jack: living with the all-clear

Paul Linsley

Understanding Jack's concerns

I am visiting Jack at home in my capacity as a community mental health nurse following a referral from his GP. My referral notes inform me that Jack is 57 and has successfully undergone treatment for prostate cancer but is struggling to adjust to being given the 'all clear' verdict and living cancer-free. Prostate cancer is the most common cancer in men in the United Kingdom (UK). The incidence has risen significantly over the past decade, with around 55,100 new prostate cancer cases in the UK every year; that is around 150 every day (Cancer Research UK, 2024). This increase is largely attributed to the greater use of Prostate Specific Antigen (PSA) testing. Despite the rising incidence, death rates have been falling owing to public awareness and screening programmes, along with advances in cancer treatments, personalised medicine and genetic testing, amongst other measures.

> *APPROACH: PSA testing*

Jack greets me at the door and rushes me into the house as if afraid the neighbours might see me. Stigma around both cancer and poor mental health is common. Once settled in his front room, I ask him to tell me a little bit about himself and his understanding of the reason for referral.

> *APPROACH: case formulation; unconditional positive regard*

'I had prostate cancer,' he explains. 'It was all very frightening, and I thought I was going to die. I had always lived what I consider to be a healthy lifestyle, and hardly ever took time off work. One day I noticed blood in my urine. I wasn't worried as I'm gay and haven't used condoms since I married my husband. I can be a little over vigorous during sex, so I just thought I might have over done it, and that I should take it a little easier. Anyway, it persisted, so I went to see my GP who then referred me to a urologist. He did a blood test and some scans to find out what the problem was. I then had a biopsy and suddenly I'm told I have cancer

DOI: 10.4324/9781003651758-8

APPROACH: radical
prostatectomy

APPROACH: radiotherapy

and that my options are surgery or radiotherapy. I opted for surgery and I'm glad to say that it was a complete success and I've been clear now for what is getting on for 8 months.'

Jack smiles uneasily before continuing, 'You'd think I would be happy and that I would be keen to get on with life, but I'm struggling with my mood, and I find that I am not the person I used to be. It's putting a strain on my husband John, who has been incredibly supportive throughout all this. He's so understanding, he really is my rock. I don't think I'd have managed without him.'

Jack takes a pause before telling me about his mood. 'I lack energy and feel drained a lot of the time, I get angry quickly and I'm snappy with people, especially with John, which is not like me at all and is unfair on him. I've started to keep things from him and find that I don't talk to him the way that I used to, which I find upsetting. I'm hesitant to talk about what's happened to me and how things have affected my body. Sometimes I struggle to get an erection. Sex is different now and it can be disappointing when things don't go to plan. I used to have a really toned body, having a physical job – I'm a mechanic and I worked out a lot. I haven't been to the gym in a while now.'

APPROACH: powerful questions

VALUE: respect and dignity

I try using powerful questions to move the assessment along and explore topics important to Jack in greater depth.

'Jack, can you tell me more about your relationship with John and how you're feeling right now?'

'It's been tough,' Jack answers. 'Things just feel different since the diagnosis. Some days, I struggle to manage my mood, and my motivation is all over the place.'

VALUE: compassion

'That sounds difficult,' I respond. 'What do you think has been the biggest challenge for you?'

Jack pauses before responding. 'Honestly? The loneliness. People expect me to just get on with my life, like everything should be back to normal. But it's not. I feel abandoned sometimes.'

Recognising the power of empathy, I reply, 'That must feel isolating. What would support look like for you right now?'

'I want people to see me for who I am, not just as a cancer survivor. I hate that label. It's as though that's all people see now, but I've always been more than my cancer,' Jack says emphatically.

'That makes a lot of sense. It sounds like you want to be recognised for all of who you are, not just for this one part of your experience. How can I support you in that?' I ask.

We explore Jack's illness-related beliefs as part of the assessment. Illness-related beliefs play a crucial role in case formulation and treatment outcomes. These beliefs encompass patients' perceptions of their symptoms, illness origins, and how the consequences of having gone through treatment are dealt with.

APPROACH: case formulation

VALUE: equity and inclusivity

Jack explains, 'Sometimes I catch myself thinking that I brought this on myself. I'm of a generation that was told that being gay wasn't natural, and that God would punish me for being homosexual. I come from a strong religious background and thought about being punished a lot. Honestly, sometimes it does feel like a punishment and that I've done something wrong, although I know that I'm a good person generally. It's only a fleeting thought, but it does upset me sometimes.'

VALUE: cultural competence and sensitivity

Proceeding with Jack's assessment, I ask about how his recovery from cancer has impacted his social functioning and relationships. This is explored through the self-concept in case formulation, in which the person explores how they are responding at a particular point in their life compared to how others might act and think in a similar situation. In this case, the situation is 'being cancer free'.

APPROACH: psychosocial support

APPROACH: case formulation

Jack suddenly becomes quite animated, firmly stating, 'I'm not cancer free. I'm still living with the side effects of the treatment.' He lifts his shirt, 'I've grown bloody boobs and a belly; I look like I'm pregnant. I dribble after peeing. I have to wipe with a tissue after finishing peeing; otherwise,

I spend a lot of time shaking it and look like I'm pulling myself off. It's really embarrassing. I can't use a public toilet anymore.'

Jack grimaces and tries to smile, but it is clear that he doesn't find the situation in the least amusing. The whole experience is clearly unsettling for him. He turns away from me and focuses his attention on looking out of the window.

'I think it was easier having the cancer, when I felt more like my old self, than living with the effects of the treatment. I really wish I could go back in time,' says Jack woefully.

Reflection

As I drive back to base, Jack's words linger in my mind: 'I think it was easier having the cancer, when I felt more like my old self, than living with the effects of the treatment. I really wish I could go back in time.' His statement unsettles me. Despite being cancer-free, he is clearly struggling to adjust, and his distress goes beyond the physical impact of treatment.

Jack spoke openly about his feelings of loneliness and abandonment, about how people expect him to simply move on. He resents being defined by his illness, finding the label of 'cancer survivor' more isolating than empowering. As a gay man, he may also face unique challenges in seeking support, especially if those around him don't fully understand or acknowledge his experiences (Moore et al., 2019).

I find myself questioning whether I did enough to validate Jack's emotions and explore what support he truly needs. Did I give him the space to express his fears without trying to 'fix' them too quickly? Could I have approached the conversation differently? His words remind me that recovery is not just about survival but also about reclaiming identity, purpose, and a sense of belonging (Hoyt and Chase-Lansdale, 2021).

As I reflect, I realise that Jack's struggle is not just about the past he longs for but the future he doesn't yet see a way into. I am unsure how best to support patients like him in navigating this complex journey.

As I reflect on my conversation with Jack, I am struck by how survivorship brings its own set of difficulties, often overlooked in healthcare. The psychological consequences of cancer are well-documented: depression, anxiety, distress, and an enduring fear of recurrence (Vyas et al., 2022). Jack's words echoed this reality, highlighting his struggle to reconcile his identity with the long-term effects of treatment.

The transition from cancer treatment to survivorship is filled with uncertainty, a factor linked to increased physical and functional impairment (Park et al., 2020). While some patients initially experience a 'honeymoon' phase after receiving the all-clear, distress levels often rise as time progresses. Many, like Jack, grapple with lingering symptoms and emotional upheaval. His frustration is evident – while cancer was no longer a physical threat, its impact on his life remains profound. His intimate relationship with John had been altered, his body no longer feels the same, and the label of 'cancer survivor' feels more like a burden than an achievement.

One of the most significant challenges Jack faced was sexual dysfunction, a common issue for prostate cancer survivors. Studies indicate that only 22% of men report sufficient erections for insertive anal sex post-treatment, highlighting the profound impact on sexual well-being (Rosser et al., 2019). For many men, sexual function is deeply intertwined with their sense of masculinity, and disruptions in this area can lead to anxiety, depression, and relationship strain (Seidler et al., 2020). Jack's experience underscored these struggles, particularly as a gay man navigating a healthcare system that often assumes a heteronormative framework. Research suggests that gay men with prostate cancer experience worse mental health outcomes, higher distress levels, and greater fear of recurrence compared to heterosexual men (Rosser et al., 2019). Jack's frustration was not just about his body but also about the lack of inclusive healthcare conversations that acknowledged his unique concerns. Gay men recovering from cancer may experience added stress due to past healthcare discrimination and a lack of culturally competent care.

Masculinity norms further complicate adjustment, as traditional ideals of self-reliance and emotional control can hinder help-seeking behaviours (Seidler et al., 2021). Jack minimises his struggles. This is a coping mechanism observed in many male cancer survivors who feel pressured to 'move on.' However, research suggests that those who adopt avoidant coping strategies experience poorer psychosocial outcomes (Groarke et al., 2020). Encouraging open conversations about emotional well-being and fostering psychological resilience can mitigate these effects. Interventions that promote mindfulness and acceptance-based approaches have shown promise in shifting the focus from erectile function to overall sexual health and intimacy (Bossio et al., 2021).

THEORY: resilience theory

Jack's journey highlighted the critical role of social support in survivorship. While gay men often rely on expansive support networks, they may also isolate themselves during treatment to avoid burdening others (McInnis and Pukall, 2020). Jack expressed feeling alone in his struggles, a sentiment linked to minority stress, internalised stigma, and body image concerns (Badenes-Ribera et al., 2018). Studies indicate that the internalisation of masculine body ideals and sociocultural pressures within the gay community contribute to body dissatisfaction and mental health struggles (Metin-Orta and Metin-Camgöz, 2018). Jack's difficulty accepting his post-treatment body reflects these broader challenges, further complicating his adjustment.

THEORY: minority stress theory

Recognising the need for additional support, I directed Jack to a local LGBTQ+ prostate cancer support group. Research highlights the effectiveness of peer support in reducing distress and improving psychosocial well-being in cancer survivors (Crawford-Williams et al., 2018). For Jack, this group became a turning point. He described it as 'a breath of fresh air,' appreciating the open and frank discussions about living and surviving prostate cancer. His husband, John, also became involved, attending meetings and contributing to conversations they previously avoided at home. Their relationship, once strained by unspoken fears and frustrations, began to heal through shared dialogue and mutual understanding.

Jack found new meaning in sharing his experiences, eventually becoming one of the group's more experienced members in discussing sexual well-being. Studies show that benefit-finding (identifying positive changes through adversity) can lead to post-traumatic growth and improved psychological adjustment (Majid and Ennis, 2018). For Jack, helping others navigate the challenges he once faced provided a renewed sense of purpose and agency.

Reflecting on Jack's journey reinforces the importance of individualised, inclusive care in cancer survivorship. Prostate cancer treatment does not end with remission; it continues in the form of long-term physical, emotional, and relational adjustments (Dunn et al., 2023). Nurses play a critical role in providing anticipatory guidance, setting realistic expectations, and addressing specific stressors to improve quality of life (Cathcart-Rake et al., 2023). Incorporating survivorship care plans that address psychosocial concerns, sexual health, and minority stress can enhance patient outcomes and satisfaction (Moore et al., 2019).

Jack's story is a reminder that cancer survivorship is not just about living. It is about finding a way to thrive despite the challenges. His resilience, shaped by support and shared experiences, illustrates the profound impact of inclusive, patient-centred care. As healthcare professionals, we must continue to foster environments where survivors feel heard, validated, and empowered to navigate life beyond cancer.

Questions for reflection and discussion

Explore the key issues raised in the above scenario as you answer the following six questions:

1. Body image, self-esteem, and masculinity are three interconnected constructs in men with prostate cancer, with profound effects on quality of life. Explore how each of these might impact a person's thinking and actions to the detriment of their well-being.

2. When thinking of adjustment following treatment, what do you think patients expect? For example, do you think that patients expect no side effects, minimal impact on quality of life, or things to be as they were? How might unrealistic expectations impact a person's well-being?

3. What strategies might Jack use to begin rebuilding his relationship with his husband, John?

4. What are the things that you value in life, and how might you stay connected with these during and following treatment for a major illness?

5. Take the time to research local support groups for individuals with and recovering from prostate cancer. Consider how you can effectively signpost patients to these and similar resources as needed in the future.

6. What access to specialist services – incontinence and sexual dysfunction clinics – do people receiving and recovering from prostate cancer have in your local area?

Further reading

Cancer Research UK: Sex and erection problems after treatment for prostate cancer. https://www.cancerresearchuk.org/about-cancer/prostate-cancer/practical-emotional-support/sex-relationships/difficulty-getting-erection (Accessed: 17th February 2025).

Prostate Cancer UK: Information for gay and bisexual men. https://prostatecanceruk.org/prostate-information-and-support/living-with-prostate-cancer/information-for-gay-and-bisexual-men (Accessed: 17th February 2025).

Kamen, C. and Lucht, M. (2020) Cancer in LGBTQ+ individuals: A review of psychosocial considerations and implications for care. *Current Oncology Reports*, 22(3): 22.

This article focuses on the psychosocial challenges faced by LGBTQ+ individuals, particularly in the context of cancer. It provides insights into mental health, stigma, and coping strategies, with a specific emphasis on how these challenges can be addressed within contemporary cancer care.

Horne, R. and George, S. (2022) Sexuality and intimacy after cancer: The experiences of gay and bisexual men. *Supportive Care in Cancer*, 30 (12): 1101–1110.

This study explores the intimate and sexual health concerns of gay and bisexual men post-cancer treatment, focusing on issues like erectile dysfunction, body image, and the role of intimacy in recovery. It provides contemporary insights into how gay men navigate sexuality and relationships after cancer.

Sileo, K. M. and Kershaw, T. S. (2021) Navigating cancer and masculinity: A qualitative study of gay and bisexual men's cancer care experiences. *American Journal of Men's Health*, 15(2), 1557988320984110.

This qualitative study examines the intersection of masculinity, sexuality, and cancer care in gay and bisexual men. It explores how masculinity norms influence their experiences with diagnosis, treatment, and post-treatment challenges. It is particularly focused on the contemporary struggles of gay men navigating both their gender and sexual identity in the context of illness.

Further information

VALUES

Compassion involves providing empathetic, sensitive care that recognises the emotional, physical, and psychological impact of both cancer and potential discrimination.

Cultural competence and sensitivity require understanding of the unique health disparities faced by LGBTQ+ individuals, including mental health considerations, higher rates of certain cancers (for example, human papillomavirus (HPV)-related cancers), and potential past negative healthcare experiences.

Equity and inclusivity involve ensuring that care is free from discrimination, biases, or heteronormative assumptions, tailoring healthcare to meet specific needs rather than a one-size-fits-all approach.

Holistic well-being goes beyond physical recovery by addressing mental health, sexual health, and body image concerns post-treatment. Encourage open discussions about sexual function, relationships, and identity after cancer.

Respect and dignity include acknowledging each patient's gender identity, sexual orientation, and lived experiences, avoiding assumptions about relationships or support systems.

THEORIES

Masculine norms play a significant role in men's behaviours and well-being. Research has identified key subjective masculine norms in the United States, including emotional toughness, providing for family, and avoidance of femininity. These norms can influence various aspects of men's lives, such as their mental health and help-seeking behaviours.

Minority Stress Theory (Meyer, 2003) explains how the stress experienced by sexual minorities due to discrimination, stigma, and marginalisation can have negative effects on their mental health and overall well-being.

Resilience Theory highlights how individuals overcome adversity, such as discrimination or illness, through personal strengths and community support (Richardson, 2002).

APPROACHES

Acceptance interventions deal with negative thoughts, feelings, symptoms, or circumstances through challenging assumptions and misconceptions relating to an event or illness.

Case formulation (CF) is a complex process that involves gathering and integrating diverse information to develop a concise account of a person's mental health problems and guide treatment. It serves as a bridge between assessment and treatment, informing psychological treatment choices. Various theoretical approaches to CF exist, including behavioural, cognitive-behavioural, psychodynamic, medical, and eclectic perspectives.

Mindfulness interventions aim to foster greater attention and awareness of present-moment experiences.

Powerful questions are a fundamental tool in counselling and coaching, serving multiple purposes. Effective counsel relies on questions to shift perspectives and deepen understanding; experienced clinicians will ask fewer but more impactful questions. Powerful questions are versatile interventions that, when applied effectively, can significantly enhance the counselling and coaching process.

PSA testing is a widely used method for investigating prostate cancer. Prostate Specific Antigen (PSA) is a protein produced by the prostate gland. The PSA test can serve multiple purposes, including screening, monitoring, and diagnosis of prostate cancer, and can be considered a public health initiative.

Psychosocial interventions combine psychological and social components to improve patient outcomes, particularly in chronic conditions like cardiovascular disease and cancer. These interventions aim to enhance patients' autonomy and community integration. They encompass various approaches, including education, behavioural training, individual psychotherapy, and group interventions. Effective psychosocial interventions are built on a trustful therapeutic alliance and shared decision-making, incorporating patients' subjective views.

Radical prostatectomy (RP) is the complete surgical removal of the prostate gland, seminal vesicles, and prostatic capsule for treating localised prostate cancer. This procedure aims to cure the disease while maintaining quality of life, but it requires a delicate balance between removing cancerous tissue and preserving nearby nerves crucial for erectile and urinary function.

Radiotherapy is a crucial cancer treatment that uses ionising radiation to destroy cancer cells. It can be delivered externally via linear accelerators, internally through brachytherapy, or systemically using radioactive substances. Treatment duration varies from 1 to 10 sessions for palliative care to 4–8 weeks for curative intent. Modern techniques like image-guided and stereotactic radiotherapy have improved accuracy and precision, aiming to maximise tumour dose while minimising damage to surrounding healthy tissues. Side effects occur due to irradiation of adjacent healthy tissues. Ongoing technological advancements, such as MRI-based systems and adaptive planning, aim to further enhance treatment efficacy and reduce toxicity.

Unconditional positive regard means accepting the person as they are, without imposing personal beliefs or societal prejudices.

References

Badenes-Ribera, L., Fabris, M.A. and Longobardi, C. (2018) The relationship between internalized homonegativity and body image concerns in sexual minority men: A meta-analysis. *Psychology & Sexuality*, 9: 251–268.

Bossio, J.A., Higano, C.S. and Brotto, L.A. (2021). Preliminary development of a mindfulness-based group therapy to expand couples' sexual intimacy after prostate cancer: A mixed methods approach. *Sexual Medicine*, 9(2). https://doi.org/10.1016/j.esxm.2020.100310

Cancer Research UK (2024) *Prostate Cancer Statistics*. https://www.cancerresearchuk.org/health-professional/cancer-statistics/statistics-by-cancer-type/prostate-cancer (Accessed 18th November 2024).

Cathcart-Rake, E.J., Tevaarwerk, A.J., Haddad, T.C., D'Andre, S. and Ruddy, K.J. (2023) Advances in the care of breast cancer survivors. *British Medical Journal*, 382: e071565.

Crawford-Williams F., March S., Goodwin B.C., Ralph N., Galvão D.A., Newton R.U., Chambers S.K. and Dunn J. (2018) Interventions for prostate cancer survivorship: A systematic review of reviews. *Psycho-oncology*, 27(10): 2339–2348. doi: 10.1002/pon.4888. PMID: 30255558.

Dunn, J., Chambers, S.K. and Ng, C. (2023). Long-term survivorship in prostate cancer: The need for individualized care and support. *Supportive Care in Cancer*, 31(3): 1121–1130.

Groarke, A., Curtis, R., Skelton, J. and Groarke, J.M. (2020) Quality of life and adjustment in men with prostate cancer: Interplay of stress, threat and resilience. *PLOS ONE*, 15 (9): 1–16

Hoyt, M.A. and Chase-Lansdale, P.L. (2021) Reclaiming identity after illness: The role of community and social connectedness in cancer recovery. *Journal of Health Psychology*, 26(2): 187–219.

Majid, U. and Ennis, J.H. (2018) The role of meaning in life in adjustment to a chronic medical condition: A review. *ECPsychology and Psychiatry*, 7.12 (2018): 1023–1030.

McInnis, M.K. and Pukall, C.F. (2020) Sex after prostate cancer in gay and bisexual men: A review of the literature. *Sexual Medicine Reviews*, 8(1): 102–110. https://doi.org/10.1016/j.sxmr.2019.08.004

Metin-orta, I. and Metin-Camgöz, S. (2018) Attachment style, openness to experience, and social contact as predictors of attitudes toward homosexuality. *Journal of Homosexuality*, 67: 528–553.

Meyer, I.H. (2003) Prejudice, social stress, and mental health in lesbian, gay, and bisexual populations: Conceptual issues and research evidence. *Psychological Bulletin*, 129(5): 674–697.

Moore, M., Batten, J. and Lazenby, M. (2019) Sexual minority men and the experience of undergoing treatment for prostate cancer: An integrative review. *European Journal of Cancer Care*, e13031.

Park, C.L., Dibble, K.E., Sinnott, S., Sanft, T., & Bellizzi, K.M. (2020). Resilience trajectories of cancer survivors: A meaning-making perspective. In *Navigating life transitions for meaning* (pp. 129–144). https://doi.org/10.1016/B978-0-12-818849-1.00008-4

Richardson, G.E. (2002) The metatheory of resilience and resiliency. *Journal of Clinical Psychology*, 58(3): 307–321. https://doi.org/10.1002/jclp.10020

Rosser, B.R., Kohli, N., Polter, E.J., Lesher, L.J., Capistrant, B.D., Konety, B., Mitteldorf, D., West, W., Dewitt, J. and Kilian, G.R. (2019) The sexual functioning of gay and bisexual men following prostate cancer treatment: Results from the restore study. *Archives of Sexual Behaviour*, 49: 1589–1600.

Seidler, Z.E., Dawes, A.J., Rice, S.M., Oliffe, J.L. and Dhillon, H.M. (2021) The role of masculinity in help-seeking behaviours among men with cancer: A systematic review. *Psycho-Oncology*, 30(5): 711–720.

Seidler, Z.E., Rice, S.M., Oliffe, J.L. and Dhillon, H.M. (2020) Masculinity and mental health after cancer: A systematic review of the impact of cancer on men's sexual health and relationships. *Psycho-Oncology*, 29(5): 845–854.

Vyas, N., Brunckhorst, O., Fox, L., Van Hemelrijck, M., Muir, G., Prokar, R.S. and Ahmed, D.K. (2022) Undergoing radical treatment for prostate cancer and its impact on wellbeing: A qualitative study exploring men's experiences. https://doi.org/10.1371/journal.pone.0279250

Case study 9
Aakifah: what's in a name?

Katherine Waterfall and Ruth Sanders

An overheard conversation

I am working in a surgical ward, where I care for multiple patients a day. I thoroughly enjoy working here because of the variety of people I meet and the surgical cases I get to experience. Overall, I feel I am a valued member of the team and that I get along well with others. Outside of work, I am chatty and boisterous; however, I tend to keep my head down here. I do not want to get a reputation as the 'loud Ghanian nurse'. Most of the staff on this ward are white, and I do not want to stick out. I know that as a Black nurse, I am more likely to be referred to the Nursing and Midwifery Council for misconduct, and my practice is more likely to be scrutinised. However, what I heard on today's shift was challenging and forced me to step outside of my comfort zone.

VALUE: self-protection

THEORY: code switching

VALUE: courage

I was caring for Liz, whom I had met the day before. Whilst I was washing her, she told me her late mother was Ghanaian, and we spent some time talking about tasty recipes for kelewele and waakye, which she remembered from her childhood.

MODEL: patient-centred care

In the bay next to us, I heard my colleague Shelly come in and begin to address her patient. The patient was a new admission to the ward, admitted following a mastectomy. I heard Shelly say:

'Hello, my dear, welcome to ward 12. If you need anything here is your bell, and here is some water but please just sip it for now. I'm afraid I can't pronounce your name – Ahh…k…ifa? I know! I'll call you Africa! I know you'll have been given some meds in recovery so I'm sure you will be ok for the rest of my shift – a strong woman like yourself! I'll be back shortly just to check your obs.'

DOI: 10.4324/9781003651758-9

I heard Shelly leave briskly, pulling the curtain across. Through the curtain I heard Aakifah clearly in pain, moaning as she tried to reach the water Shelly had placed on the bedside cabinet.

THEORY: rank dynamics

At this moment, I felt conflicted. Shelly is more senior than me, and she writes the off-duty. I was hesitant to question Shelly about her practice because I had asked her earlier today whether I could request a specific date off – my son was coming home from Manchester for his birthday. She had sighed and said she would, 'see what she could do.' I was anxious; I did not want to interfere in caring for Shelly's patient; however, I could hear she was distressed. Despite being wary of Shelly, I knew Shelly was a good nurse and would not have meant to place the water outside Aakifah's reach. I decided to see Aakifah to help her reach her water.

VALUE: professionalism

Checking the facts

APPROACH: infection control

Once I had finished my care with Liz and washed my hands, I popped my head around the curtain. Aakifah asked me whether she could have some pain relief. She said she had not taken what they had given her in recovery due to nausea. I passed her the water and clarified how her name was pronounced.

VALUE: courage

APPROACH: advocacy

Tentatively, I approached Shelly in the drug prep room. I repeated what Aakifah had told me about requiring some medication. Shelly replied,

'Oh yes… What's her name?? Akrifa?? She'll have been given something in recovery. I wouldn't worry yourself about her, these middle eastern women tend to behave like princesses! I'll go back to do her obs in an hour or so – her analgesia should have kicked in by then,' and hurried off.

THEORY: stereotyping

I felt dismissed and not listened to. I pulled out Aakifah's notes and saw on her drug chart that she had indeed declined analgesia in recovery. I attempted to find Shelly to inform her, but she was with another patient. On checking the drug chart, Aakifah had been prescribed Oramorph as required. I drew up the medication as per the prescription and went to the bedside to administer it.

A matter of integrity

When I next passed Shelly in the corridor, I informed her that on checking the chart, I'd realised that Aakifah was indeed due for some analgesia. I told her that I had administered the medication and documented it on her chart, as Shelly had not been at the desk to consult, and I felt a duty to respond to the patient's needs.

Shelly seemed put out. She sighed loudly and seemed exasperated.

'Fine... fine – but pandering to her won't make her any less demanding will it!'

I did not feel comfortable challenging Shelly directly about her stereotypical views of women of Arab descent. I knew that what Shelly was saying was a common trope that these women were akin to Arabian princesses, highly demanding – and overly complaining about minimal discomfort. But I knew this to be a harmful stereotype. I know from my personal experiences that people have ideas about Black people like me having lower pain thresholds. It made me feel uncomfortable to be in a situation that I had experienced before earlier in my career. Whilst working as a junior nurse in the emergency department, I had witnessed a Black man not being believed about his pain. The staff assumed he was an addict, only there to receive opioids – when the reality was that he was experiencing a serious sickle cell crisis. In this previous case, I had been too afraid to say anything.

I had since been reading more about anti-racism principles, being an active bystander and how to advocate for change in the clinical setting whilst also protecting yourself as a member of a minority ethnic group. I had joined a membership group called 'Equality for Black Nurses' and had been reading the latest report from the NHS Race and Health

VALUE: integrity

Observatory (RHO) earlier that week. I felt I could not let this go without raising a concern.

A difficult conversation

APPROACH: continuous professional development

I knew from the active bystander training I had completed that I needed to do something. The training had taught me five potential approaches – Direct, Delegate, Delay, Distract, and Document – with an emphasis on only intervening if you feel safe to do so. As a Black woman, I felt unable to confidently raise this with my white colleague. I was conscious of putting myself in a vulnerable position, especially as Shelly

THEORY: symbolic power

is more senior than I am. Instead, I chose to 'Delegate' and speak to the ward manager – a nurse called Aoife.

On raising my concerns with Aoife, she did recognise the importance of the issue and the need for something to change. I explained how important names are to one's identity and the emotional damage that consistently mis-

THEORY: microaggressions

pronouncing someone's name can have. I explained that I used to find Aoife's name difficult to pronounce, as it is an Irish Gaelic name – and not spelt how I would imagine

VALUE: respect

it was pronounced. However, I made the effort to learn it. Aoife told me she recognised the degree of white privilege afforded to her in this regard.

Although Aoife seemed to understand the issue, she asked what I thought the solution should be. This made me feel

THEORY: black fatigue

exhausted. I had to find a lot of courage to raise this issue with Aoife, and her asking me for a solution made me feel the burden of the incident even more greatly. Even so, I suggested a campaign on the ward. Perhaps something about name pronunciation, like a poster stating, 'If you can't pronounce my name, please ask me,' to remind staff.

Aoife liked this idea and got the ball rolling to implement it. She also asked about my active bystander training and the anti-racism course I had taken. I suggested a few reading materials.

A couple of weeks later, Aoife put up the posters in the staff room and announced that staff now had to undertake a mandatory cultural competency e-learning package. She pulled me to one side and said, 'I've done some reading – and I know we have a long way to go. But hopefully this is a starting point.' This made me feel seen and acknowledged.

APPROACH: allyship

Over the next few months, more information started circulating, and the NHS RHO Anti-Racism Framework (2024) was displayed in the staff room. I happened to be there having my lunch with Shelly and a student nurse one afternoon. The student asked Shelly about the campaign, and Shelly said;

'Oh yes! It's brilliant. Initially I was not receptive to this sort of thing. I'm not a racist! But I actually hadn't realised that I probably do hold some unconscious bias. I know now that I'm definitely not perfect and have a lot to learn – these resources have all been really helpful to me.'

THEORY: unconscious bias

It was so affirming for me to hear Shelly say this out loud. I felt like my actions had made a small difference, even though there was still a long way to go to change the culture of the ward and the NHS more broadly.

Reflections

Breast cancer affects one in ten women worldwide, but the incidence is variable across different ethnicities (Yedjou et al., 2019). It is widely acknowledged that across many areas of women's health, there are significant disparities between White and Black women (Knight, 2022), and although rates of breast cancer have fallen, Black women are more likely to be diagnosed at a later stage, which impacts their outcomes and survival rates (Office for National Statistics [ONS], 2021; Workman et al., 2023).

There is a continued need to decolonise healthcare, and despite the National Health Service being comprised of a diverse healthcare worker population, nurses from the global majority lack representation in leadership roles with poorer opportunities for progression. Black nurses continue to face challenges and discrimination when seeking career progression despite the valued contribution they give to the nursing profession (Adhikari et al., 2023). This is reflected in my work and experience of rank dynamics, which highlights the challenges and dilemmas we can face when deciding to speak up (Essex et al., 2023). As Black nurses we are acutely aware of our place in the institutional hierarchy, knowing that if attention is drawn to our differences, then this could initiate difficult conversations with colleagues in positions of power who do not share the same experiences as Black colleagues. This is reported in current research findings when discussing workplace identity. For example, a recent review (Adahikari et al., 2023) suggesting unconscious bias and social-cultural prejudice are felt towards the Black minority ethnic nursing workforce, considering them as somehow separate. The desire to fit in is strong, impacting our professional lives, and code-switching behaviour is one way in which we can ensure inclusivity in the workplace. However, it is tiring and mentally draining to be in a continual state of self-editing, conscious of feeling as though we must select how much of ourselves to inhibit to be taken seriously and be considered part of the nursing team.

Not only am I aware of this in my immediate working environment, but I am also aware of the broader discrimination within the wider nursing profession. The NHS Work Race Equality Standard (WRES) found in their 2023 report that a significantly higher percentage of global majority staff experience discrimination from other staff members, findings which appear relatively unchanged since 2025. It is known that Black nurses are four more times likely to be referred to the NMC for fitness to practice than their white counterparts, comprising sixteen per cent of all fitness to practice referrals, which is nearly double the number of Black registrants (Evans, 2021). This shows the extent to which Black registrants are disproportionately singled out, with many cases closing with no case to answer for. It is also acknowledged that Black nurses are under-represented in management and leadership roles, receiving fewer opportunities for promotion and experiencing more barriers than the racial majority (Adhikari et al., 2023). Not having effective professional role models at all levels of management from diverse populations is opposed to recommendations that health services need to represent the diversity of the communities they serve (NHS England, 2023). Health services need a diverse workforce, and considering the need for nurses from across the globe, work is needed to bridge these gaps.

Instead of hiding our differences, we need to work towards a better and more fair and balanced workplace diversity. Although the changes explored here may seem small, every action can move us towards greater workplace inclusivity as well as celebrating our differences. This, in turn, can support the promotion of under-represented nursing colleagues.

Questions for reflection and discussion

Explore the key issues raised in the above scenario as you answer the following six questions:

1. What is the difference between racism and discrimination?

2. Consider what it means to be an active bystander both in the case study above and in scenarios you have come across in practice.

3. What does allyship mean, and what steps can you take to become an ally?

4. What does the term 'microaggression' mean? Can you identify any microaggressions from this case as well as in your own practice setting?

5. What does it mean to be Anti-Racist?

6. Identify and explore steps that can be taken in your professional environment to make it more supportive of cultural differences.

Further reading

Kendi, I. X. (2019) *How to be an antiracist.* London, Penguin.

Nursing and Midwifery Council (2018) *Being inclusive and challenging discrimination.* www.nmc.org.uk/standards/code/code-in-action/inclusivity/ (Accessed 18th February 2025)

Royal College of Nursing (2024) *Equity, diversity and inclusion.* www.rcn.org.uk/About-us/Equity-diversity-and-inclusion (Accessed 18th February 2025).

Oxtoby, K. (2020) How unconscious bias can discriminate against patients and affect their care. *British Medical Journal*, 371. doi: https://doi.org/10.1136/bmj.m4152

Sowemimo, A. (2023) *Divided: racism, medicine and why we need to decolonise healthcare*. London, Wellcome Collection.

Further information

VALUES

Courage enables us to do the right thing for the people we care for and to speak up when we have concerns.

Integrity includes taking responsibility and holding oneself accountable for mistakes. Acting with integrity means being honest, with strong moral principles embedded within your practice.

Professionalism includes a variety of behaviours and values which the Nursing and Midwifery Council (2018) outlines in the Code under four themes: Prioritise people, practice effectively, preserve safety, and promote professionalism and trust.

Respect is an intentional act of showing consideration for another individual's well-being and a recognition of the value of a patient or colleague as a person.

Self-protection is the ability to respond to both physical and mental violence to protect yourself. This can include removing yourself from a situation.

THEORIES

Black fatigue is the exhaustion born of small acts of aggression a Black person endures. This includes the endless need to prove worthiness and exposure to news about injustice and racism inflicted on people who look like you.

Code switching refers to altering your 'code' or way of speaking in certain contexts, depending on whom you are speaking to. This can include changing your dialogue, body language, linguistic accent, the way you dress, or what you choose to eat or drink.

Decolonisation in healthcare refers to the process of rebuilding knowledge systems and institutions without the cultural and social impact of colonial violence, racism, and Eurocentrism. It is important in healthcare because modern health systems continue to be shaped by the entrenchment of Western scientific thinking and exploitation.

Microaggressions are defined as "The everyday verbal, non-verbal and environmental slights, snubs or insults, whether intentional or unintentional, which communicate hostile, derogatory or negative messages" (Sue et al., 2019). These disproportionately affect Black and Minority Ethnic people and can take the form of casual remarks, colour 'blindness', questions, or comments based on stereotypes and undermining others in public.

Rank dynamics is a way of describing interactions and relationships between people at distinct levels within a hierarchical system, such as those often seen in healthcare systems.

Stereotyping is the use of over-generalised beliefs about groups of people, often based on assumptions made about specific characteristics thought to be held in common by all individuals in the group.

Symbolic power: This concept accounts for the tacit domination of certain groups over others. Symbolic power accounts for discipline used against others to confirm that person's placement in a social hierarchy.

Unconscious bias is a form of social stereotyping about certain groups of people, formed outside of conscious awareness. Due to the tendency of humans to organise the social world by categorising people into groups, everyone holds unconscious beliefs about the various social and identity groups they come across.

APPROACHES

Active bystander is used to refer to an individual who actively intervenes when witnessing an inappropriate remark or event, as opposed to passively watching it unfold. There are many ways to be an active bystander, which can include distracting the perpetrator, disrupting the exchange to prevent it from escalating or directly asking the individual to stop.

Advocacy is a process through which it is ensured that every service user is heard and understood. It is an important concept in health and social care practice, sometimes being used as a way of describing the practitioner-patient relationship.

Allyship: An ally is a person with privilege and power who works in solidarity or partnership with a marginalised person or group to support them and challenge discriminatory systems.

Continued professional development (CPD) is an essential component of professional practice and a requirement of maintaining professional registration. It is comprised of various learning activities, including participatory learning alongside colleagues and the wider multidisciplinary team, mandatory training, engaging with current research related to nursing practice, and coaching and mentoring. Each qualified nurse is required to complete 35 hours of CPD for each revalidation period (NMC, 2021).

Infection prevention and control is an evidence-based approach which uses preventative measures to reduce the potential for patients and healthcare professionals to be harmed by avoidable infections (World Health Organisation, 2023).

Person-centred practice is an approach to working with people which provides dignity, respect, and choice.

Safe medication management is the effective administration of medication in a way which reduces the potential for harm or error.

References

Adhikari, R., Corcoran, J., Smith, P., Rodgers, S., Suleiman, R. and Barber, K (2023) It's ok to be different: Supporting black and minority ethnic nurses and midwives in their professional development in the UK. *Nurse Education in Practice*, 66: 103508, ISSN 1471-5953. https://doi.org/10.1016/j.nepr.2022.103508

Essex, R., Kennedy, J., Miller, D., and Jameson, J. (2023) A scoping review exploring the impact and negotiation of hierarchy in healthcare organisations. *Nursing Inquiry*, 30: e12571. https://doi.org/10.1111/nin.12571

Evans, N. (2023) Black and Asian nurses are more likely to face fitness to practise proceedings – and to have their cases dropped early. So what can be done to end the prejudice? *Nursing Standard*, 38(3). https://nmcwatch.org.uk/bias-in-nmc-referrals/#:~:text=Every%20day%2C%20on%20average%2C%20two,the%20proportion%20of%20black%20registrants (Accessed 22nd March 2025).

Knight, M. (2022) MBRRACE-UK update: Key messages from the UK and Ireland Confidential Enquiries into Maternal Death and Morbidity 2021. *The Obstetrician & Gynaecologist*, 24(1): 79–81.

NHS England (2023) *NHS England Equality, Diversity and Inclusion Improvement Plan*. https://www.england.nhs.uk/long-read/nhs-equality-diversity-and-inclusion-improvement-plan/#:~:text=%5B5%5D%20For%20example%2C%20women,to%2017.9%25%20of%20heterosexual%20staff.&text=Staff%20who%20are%20bullied%20are,and%20admit%20mistakes%5B7%5D.&text=Fair%20treatment%20of%20every%20individual,to%20avoid%20discrimination%20at%20work (Accessed 28th March 2025)

NHS Race and Health Observatory (2024) *Seven Anti-Racism Principles*. [Online]. https://www.nhsrho.org/resources/seven-anti-racism-principles/ (Accessed 18th March 2025).

Nursing and Midwifery Council (2018) *The Code* [Online]. https://www.nmc.org.uk/globalassets/sitedocuments/nmc-publications/nmc-code.pdf (Accessed 15th March 2025).

Nursing and Midwifery Council (2021) *Continued Professional Development*. https://www.nmc.org.uk/revalidation/requirements/cpd/ (Accessed 22nd March 2025).

Office for National Statistics (2021) *Mortality from Leading Causes of Death by Ethnic Group*, England and Wales. https://www.ons.gov.uk/peoplepopulationandcommunity/birthsdeathsandmarriages/deaths/articles/mortalityfromleadingcausesofdeathbyethnicgroupenglandandwales/2012to2019 (Accessed 20th March 2025)

Sue, D., Alsaidi, S., Awad, M., Glaeser, E., Calle, C. and Mendez, N. (2019) Disarming racial microaggressions: Micro intervention strategies for targets, White allies, and bystanders. *American Psychology*, 74(1): 128–142.

Workman, S., Thompson, M. and Lau, L. (2023) Decolonising medical knowledge – The case of breast cancer and ethnicity in the UK. *Journal of Cancer Policy*, 36: 100365.

World Health Organisation (2023) https://www.who.int/health-topics/infection-prevention-and-control#tab=tab_1

Yedjou, C.G., Sims, J.N., Miele, L., Noubissi, F., Lowe, L., Fonseca, D.D., Alo, R.A., Payton, M. and Tchounwou, P.B. (2019) Health and racial disparity in breast cancer. *Advances in Experimental Medicine and Biology*, 1152: 31–49. doi: 10.1007/978-3-030-20301-6_3

Case study 10
Antony: on the face of it

Sarah Housden

Antony's referral

Antony's referral describes him as a 56-year-old man whose cancer began in the oral cavity; he is experiencing depression and social isolation, alongside an altered sense of identity due to moderate changes in his appearance and speech. He is also having difficulty eating, following surgery to remove part of his tongue and lower jaw. He has had plastic surgery to mitigate some of the resulting facial disfigurement and has been referred to me as an occupational therapist for potential interventions relating to restoring his confidence in work and social settings, alongside practical and psychological preparation for further surgery which is planned for three weeks' time.

MODEL: oral cavity cancer

THEORY: disfigurement

THEORY: representation of the self

APPROACH: eating and drinking

THEORY: self-image

THEORY: occupational roles

APPROACH: psychosocial approaches

Before meeting Antony, I spend a few moments trying to put myself in his position. I ask myself what it might be like to look in the mirror and see an altered facial shape, to open my mouth to chat with friends or family and hear myself produce distorted or impaired speech, and to go to eat in front of others when I can no longer chew or swallow effectively, and, worse still, have difficulty keeping food in my mouth as I chew and have a tendency to drool whilst eating. There is little surprise that Antony has lost his confidence, and there is nothing exceptional in his referral in terms of work-related rehabilitation other than that his actual occupation has not been noted, so I am not sure at this stage how much of a challenge this might be for him.

APPROACH: empathy

VALUE: curiosity

VALUE: caring

THEORY: occupational disruption

VALUE: understanding

THEORY: purposeful activity

The computer beeps, and I see the pop-up notification telling me that Antony has arrived at the department for his appointment. My clinic is running on time, and I am keen not to keep him waiting, so I go to greet him in the waiting area.

DOI: 10.4324/9781003651758-10

Meeting Antony

THEORY: non-verbal communication

Antony is sitting at the edge of the waiting room with his head down and his gaze directed towards the floor. On hearing his name called, he gets up without looking directly at me, nods his head in recognition that I have spoken when I greet him, and walks with me down the short corridor to the consultation room. Respecting his silence, I say nothing until we reach the door of the room, where I welcome him again and offer him a seat. He sits down, without looking at me, and still doesn't speak, so I try introducing myself again.

'Thank you for coming to see me today, Antony. I'm Sandra, and I'm a specialist occupational therapist. I sometimes work with people being seen by the oncology team because there are some things which need a whole life understanding – about your roles, your job and your general wellbeing. I'll look beyond the surgery you've needed to discuss with you what impact it has had on your roles in every part of your life and how we can work together to set goals to restore some of those things, from everyday functioning at home to hobbies and paid or voluntary employment, as well as your relationships with friends and family members or any intimate relationships.'

MODEL: whole person care

APPROACH: goal setting

APPROACH: activities of daily living

I am aware that I am talking without any real sense of where I am heading now, slightly disconcerted by Antony's lack of a discernible response to what I am saying. I stop speaking, pausing for longer than is comfortable for me, to see if he needs more space and time to respond. I wonder what sort of an impression I have made so far and feel a degree of self-doubt arising as Antony still does not look at me and continues to be silent. I know it is not how I am feeling in this moment that is important. I think back to a few minutes ago when I had been empathically focused on Antony and wondering what living with changes to his appearance, body image, self-identity and everyday social functioning might be like for him. In this moment, I know that it doesn't matter how many other people with similar surgery to remove tumours from the oral cavity, head and

APPROACH: therapeutic silence

VALUE: patience

VALUE: self-awareness

VALUE: compassion

APPROACH: reflective practice

neck I have seen; none of them until now have been Antony. In this moment, with his unique experiences and feelings about his situation, his interactions, and his relationships. I remain silent, wanting to give Antony the chance to orientate to me and any support I might be able to give him, rather than me pushing my agenda on him.

MODEL: head and neck cancers

THEORY: interrupted identity

MODEL: person-centred practice

It may be only a minute, but it feels like a considerably longer time before Antony speaks. Although his speech is impaired, I clearly hear and listen attentively as he says, 'My partner has left me. We were going to get married. She says she can't see me the same way because I dribble when I eat and speak. I don't feel like a man anymore. It is literally just part of my tongue and jaw that's affected, but it's taken away my whole manhood. That surgeon may as well have gone the whole way and emasculated me. What do you make of that? She wouldn't even wait to see how things turned out. Just upped and left.'

APPROACH: active listening

THEORY: social stigma

THEORY: body image

THEORY: sexuality

He pauses for a few seconds, then continues: 'She was horrified. I saw it in her face. I don't want to see that in anyone's face again. So, you can forget your occupational this and your social that and the other. Plenty more opportunities out there for relationships, do you think? She was my life.'

I do not answer but let his words hang in the air. His voice is slightly raised and full of tense accusation. I remain focused on him. Although I am inwardly alarmed by the intensity of his anger, I nonetheless feel compassion and some degree of understanding. I recognise, though, that in reality I am not standing in his shoes – I am just imagining what it might be like to do so. I am keen to demonstrate unconditional positive regard and acceptance towards Antony now, hopeful that this will make a difference to how he sees himself going forward. His story and experience are unique to him, and yet, there is something in the raw intensity of the distress and sense of loss he expresses in this brief interaction that he is likely to share with so many other people with similar appearance-altering cancers.

VALUE: respect

APPROACH: unconditional positive regard

APPROACH: realism

VALUE: acceptance

THEORY: self-concept

An identity in conflict

My role as a fellow human being and as a therapist involves seeking to understand and support Antony beyond this moment of doubting his identity, worth, and masculinity to such an extent that he is encountering this critical peak of emotional crisis and expression. I am therefore keen that he knows that I respect him for sharing his fears about what the future will hold and his experience of rejection by his partner. I also want him to be able to maintain his self-respect and sense of dignity, which could be central to retaining and regaining a strong sense of self.

THEORY: self-respect

With further surgery planned for three weeks' time, I need to work with him to restore his confidence that it is worthwhile going through this further medical procedure, with its associated physical and psychological discomfort, and the subsequent adjustment to eating, speaking, and swallowing.

VALUE: collaboration

APPROACH: rehabilitation

'Antony' I begin: 'I hear your distress. I can't say that I have ever experienced anything like it myself, but I have worked with many men and women who have sat where you are and have, in time, come to see things in a new light. That does not in any way detract from the distress and loss you are experiencing now. The truth is, I can't promise you that the intensity of this distress and the fear of the future you may be feeling right now will ever diminish. But what I can tell you is that rather than moving on or being in denial of what is happening, you can expand your sense of self to accommodate these difficult changes in your life circumstances.'

VALUE: honesty

THEORY: self-identity

VALUE: hope

I pause and wait for Antony to respond. After a moment, I notice that he is lifting his head and turning his face in my direction. I feel hopeful that something of what I am saying has the potential to give him some hope that although life will not be the same again, that does not mean that it will not be worth living.

THEORY: quality of life

It is essential that we find a way forward together and that I can support Antony to understand and prepare for the nature of the changes he will face if he chooses to go

APPROACH: shared decision-making

ahead with the forthcoming surgery. At the same time, I recognise that the risks associated with delaying treatment because of his fear of further disfigurement or the social stigma of this and the difficulty of adjusting psychologically to significant changes in appearance which may impact on his longer-term chances of survival.

THEORY: patient choice

THEORY: social identity

APPROACH: self-management

The close association between an individual's personal identity, their appearance and the impact of their resulting self-perception, and so on their will to live, has never seemed so crucial in supporting a patient to make decisions about planned surgery. My professional role in this moment is to help Antony move to a point of being able to conceive of a future in which his current losses are part of his experience, rather than the most important dimension of his life story.

VALUE: courage

Antony is looking at me, so I continue: 'You see Antony, what you are experiencing is similar to the loss experienced following a bereavement. When we have to let go of someone through death, we don't forget that person, and neither is it necessarily helpful to try to forget them. In fact, the experience of loss, whatever the cause of that loss, becomes part of who we are as we carry on living. You don't have to forget your partner or your old self. But there will be ways in which you need to adjust to changes in your appearance and in how you go about some aspects of everyday life.'

VALUE: communication

THEORY: loss

THEORY: adjustment to change

I pause to check that Antony is still following what I am saying and to give him a chance to respond. He nods, so I continue: 'There are many unknowns in what lies ahead, but we can work together with others to make eating, drinking and speaking somewhat easier, and to support you as you adjust to those changes which are likely to happen.'

Antony has been silent but attentive for some minutes. He now looks directly at me and asks, 'When do we start?'

'I think we already have, Antony,' I reply, knowing that although the journey of recovery and rehabilitation from further face and mouth surgery will have many challenges, Antony's willingness to see things differently and his ability

APPROACH: multidisciplinary
team

to expand his self-concept to embrace change will make this journey a slightly easier one for Antony and the entire team.

Reflections

The way in which cancer can disrupt participation in everyday activities suggests a natural place for occupational therapy as a key approach to preparing for and recovering from treatment. However, it is helpful to be aware of the nature, scope, and supporting evidence for the occupational therapy role across all stages of the disease trajectory (from diagnosis to recovery to palliative care) and across the lifespan.

Cancers of the head and neck (HNC) are a heterogeneous group of cancers occurring in cosmetically and functionally critical areas of the body and can lead to life-altering disfigurement, as well as difficulty swallowing and speech problems. Patients with HNC are more than twice as likely to die by suicide as other cancer patients (Osazuwa-Peters et al., 2018). Elements contributing to this include the way in which a person's face plays a key part in the expression of their personality, self-image, and engagement in relationships. A further consideration is that the face is, in many cultures, the most exposed part of the body, which conveys individual identity and represents the self, whilst also being central to communication and the expression of emotions.

Combining psychological therapies with cosmetic treatments following HNC is important in preventing the development of psychological ill-health and highlights the complexity of shared decision-making, which requires discussion between patients and clinicians at every stage of diagnosis and treatment.

Questions for reflection and discussion

Explore the key issues raised in the above scenario as you answer the following six questions:

1. What professional, personal, and emotional challenges might you and your colleagues experience when working with people with facial disfigurements?

2. In the context of facial disfigurement following surgery for mouth cancer, why might it be legitimate to support people to seek social goals beyond the pursuit of improving their personal appearance as part of adjusting to their new reality and a new self-identity?

3. Identify how you and your colleagues can incorporate assessment for social well-being, alongside anxiety and depression as priorities affecting well-being and quality of life, into your everyday work with people living with cancers affecting body image and self-identity.

4. Explore ways of working with occupational therapists and other professionals to identify threats to social and occupational functioning where cancer has an impact on the concept of the self.

5. Discuss ways in which eating and drinking are fundamental to everyday psychological, social, spiritual, and community well-being, alongside their role in ensuring the consumption of adequate nutrition.

6. What types of impact are acquired facial disfigurement and alterations to body image likely to have on different dimensions of quality of life – including sexuality and social functioning?

Further reading

The following Open Access journal articles provide insight into contemporary understandings and research findings around body image, self-esteem, and quality of life in patients experiencing changes to the head, face, and oral cavity due to cancer or cancer-related treatments. Together these articles emphasise the life changing nature of the impact of these cancers and clarify the need for a multi-professional team approach.

Covrig, V.I., Lazăr, D.E., Costan, V.V., Postolică, R. and Ioan, B.G. (2021) The Psychosocial Role of Body Image in the Quality of Life of Head and Neck Cancer Patients. What Does the Future Hold? – A Review of the Literature. *Medicina.* 57(10): 1078. https://doi.org/10.3390/medicina57101078

Matsuda, Y., Jayasinghe, R.D., Zhong, H., Arakawa, S. and Kanno, T. (2022) Oral Health Management and Rehabilitation for Patients with Oral Cancer: A Narrative Review. *Healthcare.* 10(5): 960. https://doi.org/10.3390/healthcare10050960

Palitzika, D., Tilaveridis, I., Lavdaniti, M., Vahtsevanos, K., Kosintzi, A. and Antoniades, K. (2022) Quality of Life in Patients with Tongue Cancer after Surgical Treatment: A 12-Month Prospective Study. *Cureus.* 14(2): e22511. doi:10.7759/cureus.22511

Tonsbeek, A.M., Hundepool, C.A., Roubos, J., Rijken, B., Sewnaik, A., Verduijn, G.M., Jonker, B.P., Corten, E.M.L. and Mureau, M.A.M. (2024) Quality of Life in 583 Head and Neck Cancer Survivors Assessed with the FACE-Q Head and Neck Cancer Module. *Oral Oncology.* 153: 106813, ISSN 1368-8375, https://doi.org/10.1016/j.oraloncology.2024.106813

Wojtyna, E., Pasek, M., Nowakowska, A., Goździalska, A. and Jochymek, M. (2023) Self at Risk: Self-Esteem and Quality of Life in Cancer Patients Undergoing Surgical Treatment and Experiencing Bodily Deformities. *Healthcare.* 11(15): 2203. https://doi.org/10.3390/healthcare11152203

Further information

VALUES

Acceptance is central to person-centred practice. It sits alongside being non-judgemental and understanding the perspective of the person as a central tenet of working with people living with cancer as they present throughout their illness trajectories. It is key to promoting patient well-being.

Caring involves practitioners engaging in interactions and interventions which focus on the needs of the person within their context. Caring also includes making use of an evidence-based approach to providing the right care, in a timely way, at every stage of life.

Collaboration with patients as well as with colleagues is an essential aspect of providing high-quality care, as each professional brings unique skills and tools to the team. (See also **multi-disciplinary team**).

Communication is 'central to successful caring relationships and to effective team working. Listening is as important as what we say and do' (Department of Health, 2012, p. 13).

Compassion is defined in Compassion in Practice as 'how care is given through relationships based on empathy, respect and dignity' (Department of Health, 2012, p. 13).

Courage is described within compassion in practice as enabling 'us to do the right thing for the people we care for, to speak up when we have concerns and to have the personal strength and vision to innovate and to embrace new ways of working' (Department of Health, 2012, p. 13). It is helpful to note that patients as well as practitioners require courage to navigate the cancer journey.

Curiosity involves going beyond what is immediately obvious by observing, listening, asking questions, and reflecting on the information gathered.

Honesty is an essential quality in any person working in healthcare due to the vulnerability of service users, many of whom will be living with long-term illnesses or conditions, which may make them fully or partially dependent on the care and support of others.

Hope has been described as an integral part of being human and is seen as having three main dimensions: firstly, an inner power that enables people to transcend their present situation; secondly, the anticipation of an improved state; and lastly, as a personal experience centred on our chances of achieving what we want (Antunes et al., 2023).

Patience is an essential ingredient to avoiding outpacing the people with whom we work. We need to adjust the pace of both speech and action to that of the person with whom we are working. This is a key aspect of person-centred practice.

Respect involves recognising and acknowledging the unconditional value of people in a way which enables them to maintain their dignity and self-respect.

Self-awareness of practitioners providing health and care services is integral to reflective practice, delivering person-centred practice, and the therapeutic use of self to build relationships focused on a shared understanding of things which are important to the patient.

Understanding involves having a sympathetic awareness of another person's thoughts, feelings, and experiences and is central to providing person-centred practice, as well as to providing approaches which help to avoid stress and distress for patients of all backgrounds and abilities.

THEORIES

Adjustment to change is an essential aspect of avoiding undue stress in the face of a cancer diagnosis. Within themselves, diagnosis of and treatment for cancer require an ongoing process of change as the condition progresses or improves. Being unable to adjust or to adopt new responses to changed living situations, environments, or contexts of care can exacerbate stress and distress for the person living with or surviving cancer.

Body image can be defined as a person's internal picture of what their own body looks like. For some people, this will be closely connected to their social confidence, sense of self-esteem, and self-identity.

Disfigurement is a medical term which reflects the idea of a significant change to appearance in a way which detracts from a person's external beauty. A disfigurement may exist from birth or can be acquired and is linked strongly to Erving Goffman's (1963) concept of social stigma.

Interrupted identity is a form of identity disturbance which can lead to quite marked and noticeable changes in self-image, conveyed by changing goals, values, and aspirations.

Loss of any kind can be accompanied by a grief response and does not necessarily involve the death of a person close to us. Loss and grief can also be experienced because of losing contact with an important person, object, stage of one's life or other significant change, such as the diagnosis of a life-limiting illness, as occurs in some cancers. The grief experience has been described as involving five stages of processing loss (Kubler-Ross and Kessler, 2014), although this model has been both built upon and contested by other authors.

Non-verbal communication includes gestures, facial expressions, movements, muscle tension, and posture, alongside the volume, tone, and pitch of vocalisations. Each person has an individual profile of non-verbal communication, although there may be some culturally and socially derived gestures and expressions which people from similar backgrounds share.

Occupational disruption occurs when there is an abrupt change in a person's routine and engagement in meaningful occupations due to factors beyond their control, which may harm their health and well-being (Nizzero et al., 2017).

Occupational roles refer to the responsibilities and tasks individuals have in their work and, as such, constitute a set of norms and expectations which apply to a person's actions when carrying out a job.

Patient choice should be facilitated in all circumstances, with appropriate and full information being provided to enable an informed choice.

Purposeful activity can include any activity which has personal meaning for a group or individual or is one which aims to achieve or contributes towards achieving an established goal.

Quality of life can be difficult to define, as it is subjective, with each person having different expectations about the comfort in which they should live. The World Health Organisation defines quality of life as a person's perception of their well-being in relation to the fulfilment of personal goals and expectations (World Health Organisation, 2012).

Representation of the self includes how people picture themselves as well as how they depict themselves to others. It is likely to be disrupted or threatened in situations where physical changes occurring in cancer and other illnesses or long-term conditions lead to changes in body image and associated social functioning.

Self-concept refers to the image we have of ourselves and of the way we relate to others, including our interpretation of our actions in relation to others and how we think others perceive these.

Self-identity is the identity an individual forms about themselves, which can be affected by the social groups to which they belong, as well as by their self-esteem and roles played in wider society.

Self-image is made up over time and consists of our perceptions of the self, which can be positive or negative.

Self-respect involves having a positive sense of ourselves, which leads to a sense of confidence and liking in both how we view and feel about ourselves as individuals and in our relationships with those around us.

Sexuality involves psychological, physiological, behavioural, and social aspects of how people experience and express themselves sexually, including their emotions, attractions, and identity.

Social identity is part of a person's self-concept and thus part of how they see themselves. Social identity can be based on characteristics which give a person a sense of belonging to a group, such as race and ethnicity, gender, religion, sexual orientation, socioeconomic status, work role, and political affiliation. Where occupational or social roles are potentially threatened or disrupted due to cancer, social identity can also be disrupted.

Social stigma refers to conditions or situations which are seen as a social disgrace, as outlined by Erving Goffman (1963). Goffman considered that stigma is an attribute that extensively discredits an individual, reducing him or her from someone seen as a whole person to someone seen as being tainted, who is discounted for the label that makes them stand out from others.

APPROACHES

Active listening is an essential aspect of respecting patients. Becoming an effective listener involves actively engaging with people to make sense of what we see in their body language, in combination with what we hear. We need to hear, consider, and process what is said to us in healthcare, and this is never a passive process (Ali, 2018).

Activities of daily living (ADL) include all daily tasks and activities which contribute towards the well-being of the person. These activities can relate directly to personal care and maintaining health, domestic chores, exercise, and having periods of rest and leisure, as well as to activities which contribute indirectly to the fulfilment of wider goals – such as going shopping, using a computer, and texting or phoning friends.

Eating and drinking are everyday occupations which, as well as having a role in maintaining physical well-being, hold social and cultural meanings which are unique to individuals and social groups.

Empathy is essential for providing person-centred care. It enables the person providing support to better understand the world from the perspective of the patient and, therefore, to respond to their experience of service delivery with an individualised approach.

Goal setting should take a collaborative and person-centred approach, with documentation showing how people and their representatives of choice are supported to be involved in developing and reviewing progress towards establishing and meeting personally meaningful goals.

Multidisciplinary team working involves more than working alongside health practitioners from other professions or at a different stage of their careers. It also provides opportunities for taking into consideration different professional perspectives of relevance to decision-making, positive risk-taking and reflection on and in practice to improve patient outcomes.

Psychosocial approaches are an excellent complement to biomedical approaches and help to ensure a more person-centred approach to meeting the needs of the whole person.

Realism is a key part of providing effective and evidence-based healthcare provision for practitioners. It involves a combination of acceptance of things as they are, combined with being prepared to work to improve the situation. For patients and their families, realism helps to avoid the depressive effect of negative rumination, which can lead to catastrophising, whilst deterring disappointment which may occur through unrealistic hopes of avoiding facing the true situation.

Reflective practice: The NMC and HCPC require reflection as part of the process of maintaining up-to-date and safe practice. A range of reflective models can be used to support the process of reflection.

Rehabilitation involves regaining strength and function which may have been lost following illness or medical treatment, as well as finding new ways to approach activities or use equipment where adaptations are necessary for regaining independence in the short or long term.

Self-management is a key aspect of encouraging patient well-being and recovery in the long term. First steps to self-management are facilitated through shared decision-making and collaborative goal planning.

Shared decision-making focuses on including patients in all decisions about their own lives so that their voices are heard and their individual preferences understood and fully represented in any decision-making process which takes place.

Therapeutic silence allows time, space, and capacity for cognitive patients to process and respond to information that has been provided. Silence can offer valuable thinking time for changing perspectives and should be welcomed as an opportunity to support the person and reflect on the preceding interaction.

Unconditional positive regard involves accepting and respecting people regardless of whether you agree with their perspective, their actions or what they say. It is a respect bestowed on people primarily in recognition of shared humanity. Unconditional positive regard is a key aspect of person-centred theory as proposed and practised by Carl Rogers (in Suhd, 1995), stating that positive regard enables our service users to feel respected and valued within the therapeutic relationship. He considered that every individual develops a view of themselves which arises from interacting with people who play important roles in their childhoods. If people experience being loved, valued, and respected, they feel worthy of love, value, and respect (see Chapman, 2017, for further information on utilising person-centred care in contemporary nursing practice).

MODELS

Head and neck cancer (HNC) is a relatively uncommon form of cancer, although there are more than 30 areas within the head and neck where cancer can develop. Mouth cancer is the most commonly occurring HNC.

Whole person care involves responding to the needs and strengths of the whole person, including influences on their physical, social, psychological, and spiritual well-being, both now and in the past, whilst embedding the principles of person-centred care into every intervention.

Oral cavity cancer (OCC), also known as mouth cancer or tongue cancer, is a malignant tumour that develops in the mouth, lips, or upper throat.

Person-centred practice is an approach to working with people which provides dignity, respect, and choice.

References

Ali, M. (2018) Communication Skills 5: Effective listening and observation. *Nursing Times* [online]. 114(4): 56–57.

Antunes, M., Laranjeira, C., Querido, A. and Charepe, Z. (2023) "What do we know about hope in nursing care?": A synthesis of concept analysis studies. *Healthcare* (Basel). 11(20): 2739. doi: 10.3390/healthcare11202739. PMID: 37893813; PMCID: PMC10606526.

Chapman, H. (2017) Nursing theories 1: Person-centred care. *Nursing Times* [online]. 113(10): 59.

Department of Health (2012) *Compassion in Practice; Nursing, Midwifery and Care Staff; Our Vision and Strategy*, London: Gateway reference 18479.

Goffman, E. (1963/*1990*) *Stigma: Notes on the Management of Spoiled Identity*, London: Penguin.

Kubler-Ross, E. and Kessler, D. (2014) *On Grief & Grieving: Finding the Meaning of Grief through the Five Stages of Loss*, London: Simon and Schuster.

Nizzero, A., Cote, P. and Cramm H. (2017) Occupational disruption: A scoping review. *Journal of Occupational Science*. 24(2): 114–127. https://doi.org/10.1080/14427591.2017.1306791

Osazuwa-Peters, N., Simpson, MC., Zhao, L., Boakye, E.A., Olomukoro, S.I., Deshields, T., Loux, T.M., Varvares, M.A. and Schootman, M. (2018) Suicide risk among cancer survivors: Head and neck versus other cancers. *Cancer*. 124: 4072–4079. https://doi.org/10.1002/cncr.31675

Suhd, M.M. (1995) *Positive Regard: Carl Rogers and Other Notables He Influenced*. Palo Alto, CA: Science and Behavior Books.

World Health Organisation (2012) *The World Health Organization Quality of Life (WHOQOL)*. https://www.who.int/toolkits/whoqol (Accessed 24th December 2024).

Case study 11
Paul: a fearful decision

Louise Grisedale and Emma Harris

Paul's referral

A referral for Paul, aged 58, has come into our hospital specialist palliative care team overnight. It indicates that Paul has been admitted to the acute respiratory ward with increased shortness of breath and severe pain. He has recently been diagnosed with stage four lung cancer and has been undergoing chemotherapy and radiation therapy to treat his cancer. As the disease has progressed, Paul has experienced intense pain that has impacted on his daily activities and quality of life. His medical team has now recommended the use of opiate medication to manage his pain, but Paul is hesitant to take opiates due to fear of addiction and other side effects.

As the specialist palliative care nurse overseeing the triage of referrals this morning, I review Paul's case. The process of triaging involves reviewing each new referral to decide which member of the team would be best suited to respond, depending on the patient's needs. I follow the triage process and categorise the referrals into category one – urgent and to be seen within 24 hours (anyone with uncontrolled symptoms); category two – to be seen within 48 hours (for assessment and support); and category three – to be seen as soon as possible (assessment and signposting if required). Paul is a priority one patient due to his acute symptoms, so I set off to see him as the first on my list of patients for the day.

APPROACH: prioritisation

APPROACH: clinical judgement

Pauls' story

As I approach the respiratory ward, I mull over what I might expect. I am particularly concerned about how Paul is coping with his current pain levels.

Before going to see him, I review Paul's medical notes to find out more about his clinical history, diagnosis, and any relevant information about prognosis, medical or social history, and treatments, as well as any expressed wishes for the future. I also ask Jane, the nurse assigned to care for Paul, to update me about his referral to the palliative care team.

Jane fills me in briefly: 'Paul had a sleepless night due to shortness of breath and pain. He is not keen to talk about his condition, so it would be helpful if you can give us some guidance on how best to approach this.'

Meeting Paul

MODEL: history taking

APPROACH: communication

APPROACH: 'Hello, my name is ... campaign'

Clarity of information is essential to generate an overarching and in-depth understanding of Paul's situation and of his outlook. I approach his bed to introduce myself and explain the purpose of my visit. Smiling warmly, I begin, 'Good morning, Paul, I'm Poppy, a nurse from the specialist palliative care team. I have been asked by your consultant Mr Jones to spend some time with you, to see whether I can help? I can provide a range of support with symptoms, someone to talk to, as well as support for you and your family with planning for the future. I hear you have had a rough night.'

APPROACH: explanation of role

APPROACH: informed consent

I explain my role as part of enabling Paul to understand the reason for his referral to my team. As patients in acute settings meet numerous health professionals, it is important to explain roles, especially as some people may have concerns that a referral for specialist palliative care may mean that they are close to dying.

THEORY: non-verbal communication

Paul looks tired but maintains eye contact and seems relaxed, possibly because he has recently taken some analgesics. He sighs, 'It would be good to talk to someone about my pain, although it's not so bad now that I've had some more painkillers.'

'Would you like to go somewhere private to talk, or would you prefer to stay here?' I ask, keen to offer him as much choice and control as possible. Paul indicates that he is happy to stay at his bedside.

VALUE: privacy and dignity

I begin asking Paul for his perspective: 'Could you tell me a bit about yourself and your illness, please? Take your time, and if you want to stop at any point, just say. If there is anything that you don't understand or anything I say that you need clarity about, you can stop me. Please feel free to ask questions, and remember, I can come back later to talk again or to meet your family, if you'd like me to.'

I am interested in establishing Paul's understanding of his illness to ensure he has the knowledge needed to make informed decisions about his treatment and care. I aim to quickly develop a rapport with Paul, adopting an open posture, actively listening, allowing silences and using open questions, alongside verbal and non-verbal communication skills. I follow a structured consultation approach which enables a holistic assessment. Paul appears to feel at ease talking about himself and his family, expressing a clear understanding of his illness, diagnosis, physical symptoms, personal beliefs, and how he is coping emotionally.

APPROACH: clinical decision-making

APPROACH: communication

MODEL: Calgary Cambridge

MODEL: biopsychosocial model

I listen and ask for further information. 'Paul, you were saying that one of your main concerns is your pain. Could you describe it to me, please?' Paul points immediately to the right side of his chest under his nipple, saying, 'It's intense and there's no let up! It really hurts if I take a deep breath, and coughing and laughing make me breathless.'

I gently enquire, 'If I ask you to visualise a scale of 0 to 10, where 0 is no pain and 10 is the worst possible pain, what would yours be?'.

MODEL: numerical pain-rating scale

He looks thoughtful for a moment, 'I would say eight at the moment, because the pain feels deep in my chest and ribs, but it gets closer to 10 if I move.' It sounds like the pain originates in the intra-thoracic region. The medical notes support this, describing a 10-cm tumour with histology confirming stage 4A (IV-A) non-small cell lung cancer with the tumour infiltrating into his ribs and right lung.

APPROACH: diagnosis

I ask Paul for further detail, 'Can you tell me what helps the pain and what makes it worse?' Paul grimaces and pauses, thinking. 'Movement and coughing make it worse. Positioning with pillows helps slightly. The pain keeps me awake at night. I can't eat; I think I've lost a stone over the last month. I haven't been able to leave the house or do any work for six weeks.'

APPROACH: activities of daily living

Paul's description gives me a better understanding of how his pain affects him physically and emotionally. Cancer pain is sometimes identified as 'total pain', presenting with physical, psychological, social, and spiritual components. A multidisciplinary holistic assessment is needed to address each aspect of pain. I am keen to help to control Paul's pain so that he can enjoy his remaining time with the people close to him.

THEORY: total pain

APPROACH: holistic assessment

APPROACH: person-centred care

'Paul, I can see you are getting tired. Are you still okay for me to continue? I want to look at your medication regime and see how I can help you.'

'Yes, please Poppy.' I look at Paul's medications on the Electronic Prescribing and Medicines Administration (ePMA) system. Paul is on regular paracetamol and oral morphine sulphate when required. I ask him to tell me about his pain medications.

THEORY: ePMA

THEORY: when required medication

Hearing Paul's concerns

His reply demonstrates insight into the different types of medication: 'I find the paracetamol helps a little; it helps my general aches around my body. I know it is used for headaches usually.' The effectiveness of paracetamol is often underestimated. With its antipyretic action and fewer side effects than non-steroidal anti-inflammatory drugs (NSAIDs), it reduces fever as well as reducing the intensity of pain signals to the brain.

'I've been refusing the morphine though Poppy. I am so worried about the side effects, like addiction, and what might happen if it reduces my ability to fight the cancer. Isn't that what they give you just before you die? My daughter is getting married in a month, and I want to be mentally alert and able to walk her down the aisle.'

I wonder whether it is part of my role to convince Paul about the importance of effective pain management, to direct him in what I think is the best course of action that would give him the best quality of life from my perspective. I think it is important to explain that the intense pain he has will not go away and that we need to support him to effectively manage his pain both pharmacologically and non-pharmacologically. First, I need to see how much flexibility there is in his reservations about the use of opiates.

'Paul, I hear your concerns about taking morphine.' I pause before continuing, 'I really want to help with your pain management. Having the constant pain you are describing must be very draining, both emotionally and physically. I would like to explain how opiates work and how they react within the body. If you do get side effects, then we have ways of dealing with them and can also try alternative medications. It would be helpful to work together to reduce your concerns about the use of opiates.'

APPROACH: empathy and compassion

THEORY: adjuvant analgesic

Paul considers the information I have given him. After a few moments, I continue: 'Paul, I do understand your concerns about morphine. While it is a strong medication, we use it carefully to ensure it provides relief without causing harm. Let me explain a bit more about how we manage that. Morphine is an opioid, and it works by binding to specific receptors in the brain and spinal cord, effectively blocking the pain signals from reaching your brain. This is what provides the pain relief. What's important is that we start at a low dose, which allows your body to adjust. We will monitor you closely for side effects, such as drowsiness or nausea, and make sure we titrate the dose carefully to give you pain relief without adversely affecting your mental clarity or energy levels. Your comfort and safety are our priority, and there are always alternatives if needed.'

THEORY: pharmacodynamics

I gently ask, 'So Paul, would you consider trying a small dose of morphine to see if you experience any benefits?

MODEL: analgesic ladder

I would also add a laxative to your regular medication regime because opiates can occasionally cause constipation, and we want to reduce the chances of this happening. I'm hoping that once your pain is better managed, your appetite may come back. Eating more would give you more energy and the ability to do more. We want you to be able to walk your daughter down the aisle.'

MODEL: shared decision-making

Paul smiles, saying, 'Yes ok, Poppy, I will try it and I suppose as I'm here on the ward while I'm starting it, I can get any support I need with side effects. I do want to be in control of my own situation as much as possible though.'

APPROACH: non-pharmacological

'Paul, I'd also like us to think about some nonpharmacological interventions such as managing your shortness of breath using a handheld fan, better positioning and a referral to physiotherapy if you are happy with that.'

Paul smiles again, 'Yes please, I'm keen to get home once I am able to, so anything that might help is appreciated.'

Reviewing Paul's new medications

The next day I review Paul to see how he is feeling and to assess the effects of his new medications. 'How are you today, Paul?' I ask tentatively.

Paul's reply comes with a slightly stronger voice than yesterday: 'I had a better night and slept about six hours – the most I have slept in a long time. The nurses encouraged me to take extra morphine when the pain flared up and I was surprised how well it worked. No bad side effects either, so far.'

THEORY: when required medication

'Do you have any pain now, Paul? Like I asked yesterday, imagine if 0 is no pain and 10 is the worst possible.'

APPROACH: assessment

Without hesitation, Paul says, 'I would say three in my ribs,' and smiles.

I am relieved to hear this. 'It sounds like the morphine is working. I have looked at the amount you've had in the last twenty-four hours and calculated it to be equivalent to 40 mg.'

I continue, explaining, 'I am going to start you on a slow-release tablet of 20 mg twice a day. The aim of this is to give continual relief rather than you experiencing peaks of pain. You will of course still have the fast-acting morphine available, which we recommend you take if needed. It'll help us get the right dose for your pain. It's also useful to take that about 20 or 30 minutes before doing any activities. How do you feel about that?'

Paul contemplates this information for a moment, then smiles again and states, 'Yes, that sounds like a good plan Poppy. I feel more in control.'

'Paul, please remember to continue the paracetamol and laxatives, we may need to increase the laxative to ensure you don't get constipated. How is your breathing and appetite?' I ask, unsure of whether he will have noticed a difference yet.

Paul's voice gathers enthusiasm as he replies, 'Poppy, that handheld fan helps, the air on my face stops me feeling so panicky. And the breathing control exercises are helping too. So, my breathing feels better, and I'm eating a bit, although to be honest, I am not too worried about this. I think I will eat more when I get home to my wife's cooking.'

APPROACH: breathing control

After discussion with Paul and the clinical team, a joint decision is made to integrate the appropriate dosage and usage of opiates to include regular laxatives, with ongoing assessment of the effectiveness of the prescribed dose, which will be continuously adapted for Paul, balancing the desired effects and side effects.

APPROACH: pain assessment

My assessments, visits, and conversations lead me to believe that Paul feels listened to and in control of his own management, which is important to him.

APPROACH: autonomy

THEORY: Charter for Planning Ahead: what matters most

Furthermore, the involvement of the multidisciplinary team, such as physiotherapy and occupational therapy, complements pharmacological treatments.

APPROACH: multidisciplinary team

Ready for discharge

Paul is ready for discharge on the fourth day of his admission. I go to see him before he leaves, asking, 'How are you today? Do you and your family feel you have everything you need for going home?'

'Yes, I think so Poppy,' says Paul. 'I feel better than when I came in, so I guess that comes down to managing the pain differently. Seems like morphine is a helpful medication for me after all.'

I find myself smiling, 'I am glad we managed to get your symptoms under better control. I hope your daughter's wedding goes well. Do you mind if I just check you have everything, to make sure your discharge goes smoothly?'

Paul explains his medications to me; he is pleased that he has been reviewed by the multidisciplinary team and provided with equipment as well as breathing control advice. He is discharged home, feeling more at peace within himself, having come to terms more with his diagnosis and prognosis. He agrees to take some anticipatory medications home with him and has the reassurance that he is going to be reviewed regularly by the community specialist palliative care services.

APPROACH: discharge planning

APPROACH: 'just in case medications'

Reflections

Reflecting on the care and support I gave Paul reminds me how important it is to develop a therapeutic relationship with individual patients so that they can build confidence and trust when making important decisions about symptom control and management. Crucially, it was about providing time and information so that Paul could consider his options.

Healthcare professionals need the skills to explain the rationale for any prescription to patients and their families in terms of the chosen drug, its dosage, and any potential side effects, especially when multiple medications are prescribed.

Pain assessment, its management and the adjustment of pain medications are an essential part of reassuring Paul that he is more likely to be able to deal with other aspects of advanced cancer if his pain is well controlled. It is important to ensure appropriate medication regimes are provided for patients so that symptoms are controlled and side effects minimised, enabling a reasonable quality of life to be maintained as the end-of-life approaches.

It was important to address Paul's concerns about developing tolerance to opioids, as he is likely to require increasing doses to achieve the same level of pain relief. I explained that while tolerance can occur, the care team is experienced in managing this by carefully adjusting doses or considering opioid rotation if necessary. Paul was reassured that pain management is an ongoing process, and strategies such as adjuvant medications could be used to support his care (Pickard et al., 2020).

One of Paul's concerns was a fear that taking opioids, particularly morphine, would hasten his death. This reflects the Doctrine of Double Effect, where a treatment intended to relieve suffering (the beneficial effect) might also have a foreseen but unintended consequence, such as hastening death (Cherny and Ziff-Werman, 2023). As a palliative care team, it is essential to acknowledge Paul's fear, while also providing reassurance that the goal of opioid use is not to hasten death, but to improve his quality of life. By carefully titrating his medication and monitoring side effects, we aim to strike a balance that allows Paul to experience less pain without compromising his autonomy or causing unintended harm.

Paul was also concerned that starting on strong painkillers like morphine would signify that he was nearing the end of life. This is a common concern among patients with terminal illness, and addressing this is crucial for effective patient care. It is important for patients to recognise that pain management does not equate to giving up but instead focuses on improving quality of life and maintaining independence. As we normalise opioid use in the context of palliative care, Paul feels more comfortable starting treatment.

Paul also expressed anxiety over the potential for with-drawal symptoms should he need to stop opioids. To mitigate this concern, information about how opioids can be tapered gradually to avoid withdrawal can be provided, emphasising the importance of ongoing communication about his medication regime (Merlin et al., 2021). This can help reduce the fear of losing control over pain management in the future.

Lastly, Paul expressed concerns that opioids might affect his ability to think clearly, engage with his family, or make important decisions. To address this, we explained that while cognitive impairment can occur as a side effect of opioids, starting at a low dose and increasing gradually would help minimise these risks (Yang et al., 2023).

Although it is not explicit within Paul's case, discussions were started about Advance Care Planning (ACP), Lasting Power of Attorney (LPA), and Advance Decisions to Refuse Treatment (ADRT), each of which was followed up by the community specialist palliative care services.

Questions for reflection and discussion

Explore the key issues raised in the above scenario as you answer the following six questions:

1. How would you explain to a patient why they are experiencing pain and the different causes of pain?

2. With your understanding of pathophysiology, how would you explain to a patient how their medication is working and how each drug affects the body (pharmacodynamics)?

3. Where a person is taking multiple medications (polypharmacy), explain how you would identify and manage potential drug interactions?

4. What strategies could you use to promote effective communication when a patient and their family hold conflicting views or have different ideas about treatment decisions?

5. How can we address a patient's fear of developing tolerance to opioids while ensuring they understand how pain management will evolve over time?

6. When discussing opioid use with a patient, how would you approach the topic of balancing the need for pain relief with concerns about maintaining a clear state of mind?

Further reading

Mannix, K. (2017) *With the end in mind.* London: Harper Collins.

Mannix, K. (2021) *Listen: How to find the words for tender conversations.* London: Harper Collins.

Rabben, J., Vivat, B., Fossum, M. and Rohde, G.E. (2024) Shared decision-making in palliative cancer care: A systematic review and meta synthesis. *Palliative Medicine.* 38(4): 406–422. doi:10.1177/02692163241238384

Regnard, C. and Dean, M. (2022) *A guide to symptom relief in palliative care.* 6th edn. Oxford: Radcliffe Publishing.

Tackling Health Inequalities – Seven Priorities for the NHS (2024) https://www.kingsfund.org.uk/insight-and-analysis/long-reads/tackling-health-inequalities-seven-priorities-nhs

Further information

VALUES

Privacy and dignity – The concept of dignity has four defining attributes, including respect, autonomy, empowerment, and communication. Respect includes self-respect, respect for others, respect for peoples' privacy, confidentiality and self-belief, and belief in others. This is essential to meet individuals' needs and requirements within healthcare (Nursing and Midwifery Council, 2018).

THEORIES

Adjuvant analgesics are a small number of drugs that were approved and marketed for indications other than pain but were found to be useful as analgesics in patients receiving opioid therapy.

Charter for Planning Ahead: What matters most (2020) provides principles and questions to consider when planning for end-of-life decisions about treatment and care, useful for the public, as well as for health and social care professionals.

Drug titration is slowly increasing the dose of medications over time to minimise the risk of side effects.

Electronic Prescribing and Medicines Administration (ePMA) is software used in the NHS for electronic prescribing and medicine administration.

Non-verbal communication goes beyond the spoken word and includes gestures, facial expressions, physical appearance, and tone of voice, all of which play a part in interpersonal communication.

Pharmacodynamics is the study of how drugs interact with the body's biological systems, explaining the mechanisms through which the drug produces its effects. Pharmacokinetics is the study of how the body absorbs, distributes, metabolises, and excretes a drug. It focuses on the changes the drug undergoes inside the body.

Prophylaxis is treatment given or action taken to prevent disease or a specific known symptom.

Total pain is a theory of pain identified by Dame Cicely Saunders, who pioneered the hospice movement. It encompasses not only the physical but also the psychological, social, and spiritual dimensions of pain.

When required medication (PRN) – PRN stands for "pro re nata," which is Latin for "as needed." It refers to the administration of medication only when the patient requires it, rather than at scheduled intervals. PRN medications are commonly used for managing symptoms like pain or anxiety, which may not need constant treatment but do require intervention when they occur.

APPROACHES

Activities of daily living (ADL) include all daily tasks and activities which contribute towards the well-being of the person. These activities can relate to domestic chores, managing personal hygiene, and those that contribute indirectly to the fulfilment of wider goals, such as meeting friends socially.

Assessment is a systematic process to gather information on a person's physical, psychological, emotional, social, and environmental status. This is important for developing an accurate and holistic understanding of the patient's health condition, needs, and any potential risks.

Autonomy involves promoting the individual's ability to self-govern and their ability to make their own decisions. The NMC (2018) stresses that nurses must always promote the autonomy, rights, and choices of people in their care.

Breathing control approaches include simple measures such as keeping the room cool, using a fan, opening a window, and practising relaxation and breathing techniques.

Clinical decision-making can be based on learning from experience, critical thinking, evidence-based approaches, communication skills, teamwork, reflections, and reasoning, which together allow health practitioners to identify patients' problems and to select appropriate approaches to care and management.

Clinical judgement is a reflective and reasoning process that draws upon all available data, is informed by an extensive knowledge base and results in the formation of a clinical conclusion' (Connor et al., 2023, p. 13).

Communication is essential to build therapeutic relationships with patients – as noted by Delves–Yates (2021), you can listen without caring, but you cannot care without listening. The Nursing and Midwifery Council (2018) stresses the importance of a nurse's ability to communicate effectively and outlines related competencies that must be met to register as a nurse.

Diagnosis is identifying what is medically wrong with an individual after investigations and tests have been completed. Treatment is then planned according to the best available evidence.

Discharge planning is an interdisciplinary approach to continuity of care and a process that includes identification, assessment, goal setting, planning, implementation, coordination, and evaluation.

Empathy and compassion involve the ability to understand and share feelings, which fosters a trusting connection. Compassion demonstrates care through relationships based on empathy, respect, and dignity. Both empathy and compassion are at the heart of the NMC Code (NMC 2018, section 1.1, p. 3), which states that nurses must 'treat people with kindness, respect and compassion'.

Explanation of role is important so that patients are aware of the purpose of the healthcare professional's involvement, including their specialist skills and what interventions and support they can offer the patient.

'Hello, my Name is ... campaign' was founded by Dr Kate Granger when she was going through her cancer diagnosis and treatment. This initiative was designed to encourage healthcare staff to introduce themselves to their patients as the start of making a connection, helping patients to relax and to build trust.

Holistic assessment is a comprehensive and thorough means of evaluating an individual's health and well-being. This approach does not focus on physical symptoms or conditions in a reductionist way but considers the whole person and a range of aspects of their life.

Informed consent to treatment and care means a person must have the understanding to give permission before they receive any type of medical treatment, test, examination, or care. The person consenting must have the capacity to make the decision (NHS, 2022)

Just in case medications or anticipatory prescribing are medications that are prescribed in advance for individuals who are at the end of life for symptoms which they may experience. This is so that access to appropriate medications is swift, reducing unnecessary suffering (British Medical Association, 2024).

Multidisciplinary teamworking involves healthcare professionals working together in ways which make use of their profession-specific knowledge and skills to address the needs of patients (Taberna et al., 2020).

Non-pharmacological treatments are interventions which do not involve the use of medications. The goals of non-pharmacological interventions in pain management are to decrease fear, distress, and anxiety, which in turn help to reduce pain while maintaining the patient's sense of control.

Pain assessment is the process of asking an individual questions about their pain history, description, site, duration, and what makes it worse or better to understand and measure its extent and intensity.

Person-centred care is needed to ensure that a patient's wishes are at the forefront of their care as they near the end of life. The principles of person-centred care include treating people with dignity, respect, and compassion; offering coordinated care, support, and treatment; offering personalised care; and helping people to recognise and build on their strengths to enable better quality of life (The Health Foundation, 2016).

Prioritisation involves recognising what appears most urgent and commencing interventions as soon as possible to reduce the suffering or symptoms of individuals.

Symptom management includes managing such things as pain, nausea and vomiting, restlessness or agitation, and breathlessness. Providing good symptom management in palliative and end-of-life care is associated with improved quality of life as well as greater treatment adherence and may also offer survival advantages (Wilcock et al., 2020).

MODELS

Analgesic ladder – originally introduced in 1983 for cancer pain, it is a guide for healthcare professionals to provide relief for cancer pain (Anekar and Cascella, 2023).

Biopsychosocial model looks at the complete person alongside their behaviours, thoughts, and feelings. Engel (1977) is one model to consider.

Cambridge Calgary communication model is a well-known approach to teaching communication skills. This guideline has five steps to enabling more accurate, efficient, and supportive interviews, enhancing patient and professional experience, and improving health outcomes for patients (Silverman et al., 2013). The Calgary Cambridge model provides a framework to ensure all aspects of patient experience are covered from a holistic perspective, enhancing the patient relationship and supporting understanding of the patient's perspective. It promotes shared decision-making.

History taking is a key component of patient assessment, allowing healthcare professionals to have a better understanding of patients' problems and enabling the delivery of high-quality care (Fawcett and Rhynas, 2012).

Numerical pain-rating scale is a subjective tool used to help individuals describe the intensity of pain. This simple tool helps healthcare providers understand the severity of a person's pain and can help determine an appropriate treatment plan. It is quick to use: 1 represents very mild pain, 2 or 3 indicates mild pain, and 8, 9, and 10 most extreme pain.

Shared decision-making is a collaborative process in which patients and their healthcare providers make healthcare decisions together, considering the best scientific evidence as well as the patient's values and preferences. The patient's role in making decisions will vary from person to person (Choosing Wisely UK, 2019; NICE, 2019).

References

Anekar, A. and Cascella, M. (2023) *WHO analgesic ladder*. StatPearls Publishing [Online]. Available at: WHO Analgesic Ladder - StatPearls - NCBI Bookshelf (Accessed: 14th February 2025).

British Medical Association (2024) *Anticipatory prescribing for end-of-life care* [Online]. Available at: https://www.bma.org.uk/advice-and-support/gp-practices/prescribing/anticipatory-prescribing-for-end-of-life-care (Accessed: 10th October 2024).

Charter for Planning Ahead (2020) *What matters most* [Online]. Available at: https://www.whatmattersconversations.org/2020-charter (Accessed: 17th October 2024).

Cherny, N.I. and Ziff-Werman, B. (2023) Ethical considerations in the relief of cancer pain. *Support Care Cancer*, 31, 414. https://doi.org/10.1007/s00520-023-07868-3

Choosing Wisely UK (2019) *Shared decision making* [Online]. Available at: https://www.choosingwisely.co.uk/shared-decision-making-resources/ (Accessed: 17th October 2024).

Connor, J., Flenady, T., Massey, D. and Dwyer, T. (2022) Clinical judgement in nursing – an evolutionary concept analysis. *Journal of Clinical Nursing*, 32: 3328–3340.

Delves–Yates, C. (2021) *Beginner's Guide to Reflective Practice in Nursing*. London: Sage Publications.

Engel, G.L. (1977) The need for a new medical model: A challenge for biomedicine. *Science*, 196, 129–136. http://dx.doi.org/10.1126/science.847460 (Accessed 14th February 2025).

Fawcett, T. and Rhynas, S. (2012) Taking a patient history: The role of the nurse. *Nursing Standard*, 26(24): 41–48.

Merlin, J.S., Khodyakov, D., Arnold, R., Bulls, H.W., Dao, E., Kapo, J., King, C., Meier, D., Paice, J., Ritchie, C. and Liebschutz, J.M. (2021) Expert Panel Consensus on Management of Advanced Cancer–Related Pain in

Individuals With Opioid Use Disorder. Available at: https://doi.org/10.1001/jamanetworkopen.2021.39968 (Accessed 9th October 2024).

NHS (2022) Overview-Consent to treatment. Available at: https://www.nhs.uk/tests-and-treatments/consent-to-treatment/ (Accessed 30th June 2025).

NICE (2019) *Pain assessment* [Online]. Available at: https://cks.nice.org.uk/topics/palliative-cancer-care-pain/management/assessment-of-pain/ (Accessed 10th October 2024).

Nursing and Midwifery Council (2018) *The code* [Online]. Available at: https://www.nmc.org.uk/globalassets/sitedocuments/nmc-publications/nmc-code.pdf (Accessed 15th March 2023).

Pickard, J., McDonald, E. and Hindmarsh, J. (2020) Opioid use in palliative care: Selection, initiation and optimisation. Available at: https://pharmaceutical-journal.com/article/ld/opioid-use-in-palliative-care-selection-initiation-and-optimisation (Accessed: 24th September 2024).

Silverman, J., Kurtz, S. and Draper, J. (2013) *Skills for Communicating with Patients*. Milton: Taylor & Francis Group.

Taberna, M., Gil Moncayo, F., Jané-Salas, E., Antonio, M., Arribas, L., Vilajosana, E., Peralvez Torres, E. and Mesía, R. (2020) The multidisciplinary team (mdt) approach and quality of care. *Frontiers in Oncology*, 10: 85.

The Health Foundation (2016) *Person-centred care made simple. What everyone should know about person-centred care* [online]. Available at: https://www.health.org.uk/sites/default/files/PersonCentredCareMadeSimple_0.pdf (Accessed 26th February 2025).

Wilcock, A., Howard, P. and Charlesworth, S. (2020) *Palliative Care Formulary (7th edition)*.

Yang, Y., Cui, M., Zhao, X., Wang, S., Wang, Y. and Wang, X. (2023) Association of pain management and positive expectations with psychological distress and spiritual well-being among terminally ill cancer patients admitted to a palliative care unit. *Biomedical Central (BMC) Nursing*, 22: 96.

Case study 12
Priya: what a relief!

Louise Grisedale

The role of a community pharmacist in cancer care

Working as a community pharmacist with a background as a specialist cancer information pharmacist at a high street chemist, I often have the privilege of supporting patients through the various stages of cancer treatment. This role involves not only dispensing medications but also providing specialist advice on managing side effects, improving patient comfort, and supporting their overall treatment journey.

THEORY: pharmaceutical care in oncology

My role gives me unique insights into the complexities of cancer care patients, especially those undergoing chemotherapy, who can face a range of physical and emotional challenges. These challenges escalate over time as chemotherapy drugs accumulate in the body, causing more severe side effects. My goal is to create a supportive environment in which patients feel empowered to manage their symptoms and make informed decisions about their care.

THEORY: cumulative effects of chemotherapy

VALUE: patient empowerment

In this context, I encounter Priya, a 45-year-old woman who is undergoing chemotherapy for stage II ovarian cancer. She has come into the pharmacy looking visibly distressed but has not immediately disclosed her condition. Like many patients, she is unaware that community pharmacists can offer more than just medication.

Meeting Priya

It is mid-afternoon, and Priya is three months into chemotherapy when she approaches the pharmacy counter looking fatigued and emotionally drained. The healthcare assistant greets her warmly, and without immediately disclosing her diagnosis and treatment, Priya asks, 'What can I buy for nausea?' She quickly adds, 'Something strong

DOI: 10.4324/9781003651758-12

please,' then averts her gaze, suggesting that she wants to avoid further conversation. The healthcare assistant, noticing her discomfort, gently inquires, 'Is the nausea medication for you? Are you feeling okay today?'

Priya hesitates, her eyes welling up with tears. She continues to avoid eye contact and whispers, 'I've been unwell for a while. The treatment is ... it's just a lot to handle.'

The assistant's concern deepens, so she suggests, 'Would you like to have a chat with our pharmacist? She might be able to help.' Priya wipes her eyes, sniffs and nods. A hint of a smile on her drained and pale face suggests she is thankful for the offer.

'Please come with me. Just through here,' says the assistant, gently showing her through to the consultation room. 'Now take a seat and the pharmacist won't be long,' she explains as she discreetly places a box of tissues close to Priya.

The assistant approaches me and explains what she has observed: 'This customer seems very distressed and I think she might need additional support. She has asked for over-the-counter nausea medication, but as she is so upset, I think there might be more to her situation than just nausea.'

Recognising the need for privacy and time, I take a moment to ensure that my team can manage the pharmacy's workload while I spend time with Priya. I enter the consultation room where Priya is wiping away tears. Sitting down, I introduce myself with a warm expression, wanting to convey my openness to understanding. 'Hello, my name is Stella and I'm the pharmacist. My assistant mentioned you might be going through some difficulties right now. Could you tell me a bit about what's been happening so that I can see how we can help?' Priya takes a deep breath and trembles slightly as she composes herself. 'I've been having chemotherapy for ovarian cancer. I've been trying to manage the side effects, but it's getting harder, and I don't know where to go for help between hospital appointments, so I just came here thinking I could buy something to stop this awful sick feeling. It's spread all over me and feels like it's taking over my life, rather than just being in my stomach.'

I nod, understanding the emotional and physical toll this journey through cancer treatment can take. 'You've been carrying a lot,' I say with genuine compassion, validating her experience. 'Chemotherapy can be overwhelming, especially as time goes on. I'm really glad you're here, and we can definitely help you manage some of these side effects.'

Understanding Priya's challenges

As Priya opens up about her chemotherapy, I listen attentively. She speaks slowly but with a certain determination. 'It's been three months, and everything seems to be getting worse.'

I respond, 'It is common for chemotherapy side effects to become more severe as the treatment progresses. The chemotherapy accumulates in your system, you see, so while the symptoms might have been mild initially, they can worsen over time. After three months of treatment, many patients start noticing more severe fatigue, nausea, and other side effects.'

I pause for a moment to check her understanding. Priya nods, so I continue: 'Chemotherapy-induced nausea and vomiting (CINV) is one of the most common side effects of cancer treatment, and managing it requires a multimodal approach.' Priya has lifted her head and is looking directly at me, listening carefully to what I say. I continue by explaining, 'We can use a combination of medication, dietary changes, and other interventions to help control this more effectively.'

Priya nods with greater assurance, and I imagine that it is a relief for her to hear that what she is experiencing is normal. Understandably, her facial expression still shows concern, which is clarified as she explains, 'I've been so nauseous lately, I can barely keep anything down, and the fatigue! It's like I can't move some days, and the taste of food is unbearable!'

We discuss her medication regime, particularly focusing on what she has been prescribed for managing nausea. Priya mentions that she has been given Ondansetron, which she takes before chemotherapy and for three days after, alongside Metoclopramide for use at home. While she found the Ondansetron effective at first, she tells me that she has noticed that after her last round of chemotherapy, her nausea returned once she finished the course.

THEORY: concordance

A dilemma in symptom control

MODEL: pharmaceutical care model

I spend a moment or two considering the options for a way forward. I'm uncertain as to whether I should recommend extending the Ondansetron prescription or consider non-pharmacological options. While extending the course of Ondansetron could help alleviate Priya's symptoms, it also risks increasing side effects such as constipation, which could cause nausea itself. I also consider whether relying solely on medication is the most suitable approach. I want to ensure Priya feels empowered to manage her symptoms in a way that best suits her needs.

VALUE: medicines safety

VALUE: patient autonomy

APPROACH: evidence-based pharmacotherapy

I explain to Priya, 'Ondansetron is effective, and it can be taken for longer if necessary. However, I think we could explore other ways to help manage the nausea alongside your current medication.' I suggest some non-pharmacological strategies, including dietary adjustments such as eating smaller, more frequent meals and incorporating ginger or peppermint, which are known for their anti-nausea properties. We discuss trying light physical activities to improve her general well-being, which may also help with fatigue, alongside ensuring good hydration throughout the day.

THEORY: non-pharmacological strategies

MODEL: biopsychosocial model

'Would you like me to speak with your GP about the possibility of prescribing a longer course of Ondansetron if these approaches are not enough?' I ask, making it clear that medication could still be an option if non-pharmacological methods are not sufficient. I am keen for Priya to be involved in the decision-making process and to try different methods to see what works best for her.

As the conversation progresses, Priya seems surprised as she says, 'I didn't realise a pharmacist could help with all of this. I thought I had to wait until my next hospital visit to talk to someone about these side effects.'

I smile warmly and reassure her, 'Many people don't realise just how much pharmacists can support them, especially when it comes to managing side effects. It's all about finding a balance that works for you - using medication when necessary but also exploring other strategies that might help you feel better.' My aim is to help Priya feel more in control of her treatment while also avoiding over-reliance on medications. 'You're not alone in this. We can work with your oncologist and GP to ensure your symptoms are well-managed and to support you every step of the way.'

Addressing additional side effects

'You mentioned fatigue,' I begin, looking at Priya with a gentle smile. 'There is a careful balance between rest and light physical activity. I know it can feel impossible when you're this tired, but sometimes, small steps can help.' I pause, seeing the doubt in her eyes, and continue, 'Research has shown that gentle activities, like walking or stretching, can help reduce the intensity of cancer-related fatigue by improving circulation and boosting your energy levels.' I notice her eyes widen slightly as if the idea of being active seems overwhelming. I soften my voice, 'Exercise can also prevent muscle loss and boost your mood, which is so important when you're going through treatment. But I completely understand how daunting it sounds.' I lean towards her a little and add, 'I'm not talking about anything intense - maybe just a short walk around your garden or a few minutes of gentle stretching in the morning. It's really about what feels comfortable to you.' Priya looks at me, still hesitant. I nod, wanting her to know that I understand. 'How about this - you start small. Try a short walk, maybe just five minutes, and see how you feel. If it's too much, you can stop. The key is to listen to your body and do what feels right. If you need to rest, that's perfectly okay too. Just take it one step at a time.' I see her nodding, and I sense a small shift in her expression, perhaps the beginnings of hope. I think to myself that it's not just about giving out information; it's about showing her that she's capable and that even small actions can make a difference.

Priya shifts in her seat, a look of frustration crossing her face. 'It's the taste, too,' she says, almost in a whisper. 'Everything tastes metallic. I can't enjoy any food, and it's so disheartening.' I feel a pang of empathy, knowing how chemotherapy can strip away the small comforts, like enjoying a meal. 'That metallic taste must be so tough,' I say, leaning in to meet her eyes. 'One thing that might help is using plastic utensils instead of metal ones. I've had other patients tell me that it makes a big difference because it reduces the metallic taste.' Priya looks surprised. 'Plastic utensils? I hadn't thought of that.' I smile gently. 'I know, it's a small change, but it can sometimes make food a bit more bearable. Also, you could try focusing on more acidic or stronger flavours by adding garlic, lemon juice, herbs, spices and marinades to your cooking. Things like citrus fruits or ginger can help mask the metallic taste. Think about adding some lemon to your water or ginger to your tea.' I see her nod, so I continue, 'It's also important to stay hydrated. Sometimes using a mouth rinse before meals can help reset your taste buds a bit.' As I speak, I think about how important it is for her to regain some control. 'I know it might take some trial and error, and it's okay if not everything works. But trying different foods and techniques could help you find something you enjoy again, even if just a little. This process, this experimenting, it's about taking back some of your control.'

Priya gives a small smile, and I feel a connection with her. I sense that she is starting to see ways she can be active in her own care. I want her to leave here feeling that she has the power to improve her situation, even in small ways. 'Let's try these things,' I say, 'and if they don't work, we can think of other strategies together. You're not alone in this.'

As our conversation comes to a close, I look at Priya with a reassuring smile. 'So, we've talked about a few things that might help,' I say, summarising the new strategies Priya can try: 'Using plastic utensils, experimenting with more acidic or stronger flavours, staying hydrated, and managing your fatigue with light exercise.' I can still see the exhaustion in her eyes, but there is also a glimmer of hope there now.

Knowing it can be overwhelming to hear so many suggestions, I emphasise that it is about taking small, manageable steps. 'Priya, I know it's not easy dealing with these side effects on top of everything else you're facing.' I meet her gaze. 'But remember, it's okay to take it one step at a time. You don't need to do everything at once. Try one or two of these suggestions and see how they feel. It's about finding what works best for you, and that can take some time, and that's perfectly fine.'

I can tell that she is still worried about the nausea, so I add, 'I'll follow up with your GP regarding extending your Ondansetron prescription if needed. It can always be adjusted as we go along. And please, don't hesitate to come back or reach out if you need more advice or support.' Priya gives a small nod, and I sense more confidence, perhaps a sense of relief. 'Thank you,' she says, her voice quiet but steady.

'You're not alone in this, Priya,' I say, my tone soft but firm. 'We're in this together. Whether it's managing your medications or finding ways to help you feel more comfortable, I'm here to support you. You can always come back to the pharmacy for further guidance or need to review anything else.'

As she stands to leave, I offer her some patient information leaflets on Chemotherapy Side Effects and Eating During Chemotherapy, which provide a summary of what we have discussed. 'These might be useful to look over when you're feeling up to it,' I say. 'But again, one step at a time. We'll figure this out together.'

APPROACH: *health literacy*

Priya smiles in a tired but genuine way, and I feel a sense of satisfaction. I know this journey is long and filled with challenges, but I am committed to making sure she knows that she has someone in her corner. Empowering her to manage her symptoms, even in small ways, is a step towards making this journey a little less daunting.

Reflections

This case highlights the significant role I play as a community pharmacist in providing holistic, person-centred care to cancer patients (McCormack et al., 2021). My encounter with Priya reinforced my responsibility to not only manage medication but also to support patients more broadly, addressing both their physical and emotional well-being. One of my dilemmas was whether to request an extension to Priya's Ondansetron prescription. While this could have managed her nausea, I had to carefully weigh the potential risks, such as increased constipation, against the benefits. This reinforced the importance of ethical decision-making, balancing symptom relief with possible side effects. For patients like Priya, controlling nausea throughout the chemotherapy cycle is critical to improving the overall treatment experience. Extending the use of antiemetic medications such as Ondansetron can help mitigate these delayed effects.

Another key takeaway from this case is the importance of interprofessional collaboration in ensuring Priya received the best possible care. By liaising with her GP and oncology team, I can ensure that my recommendations align with her broader treatment plan. I recognise that working collaboratively across healthcare roles helps to bridge gaps in care, ensuring that patients undergoing complex treatments like chemotherapy receive well-rounded and continuous support.

One aspect of this encounter was Priya's lack of awareness about the role of pharmacists in managing chemotherapy side effects. Like many patients, she did not realise she could turn to me for help with her symptoms, which made me reflect on a communication gap in healthcare. This experience reinforces the importance of raising awareness amongst patients about the role of community pharmacists, not only in dispensing medication but also in offering symptom management advice and emotional reassurance. I felt a strong sense of responsibility to empower Priya by providing her with the knowledge to access appropriate support in the future.

Priya's surprise at the breadth of my role also made me reflect on the boundaries of support offered by pharmacists. I had to navigate a fine line between offering empathetic emotional support and ensuring she received specialist care when needed. I found myself questioning whether my role should extend beyond medication advice to emotional well-being or whether I would be better off focusing solely on guiding patients towards other healthcare resources. Finding the right balance is essential; while I want to be a source of comfort, I also need to recognise when to refer patients to specialist teams for further support.

The decision between extending Ondansetron and exploring non-pharmacological strategies made me reflect on the importance of patient-centred care. Rather than simply requesting an increase in her medication, I focus on empowering Priya with practical, non-pharmacological strategies like dietary adjustments, hydration, and physical activity. By doing so, I encourage her to take an active role in her symptom management, ensuring she feels in control of her care. This reaffirms my belief that while medication is valuable, it should not always be the first or only solution, especially when non-pharmacological approaches can also be effective.

This case also reinforces the significance of symptom management in cancer care. CINV remains one of the most distressing side effects for patients, yet it is often underestimated in its impact (Gupta et al., 2020). Even with advances in antiemetic agents, many patients experience delayed nausea and vomiting, which highlights the importance of continuous, proactive management. Priya's case strengthens my understanding that a combination of pharmacological and non-pharmacological methods is often the best way to address these side effects.

Supporting Priya with her fatigue was another learning point for me. I encouraged her to consider incorporating light physical activity, such as short walks or gentle stretching, into her routine. I know from experience that exercise helps prevent muscle loss and boost mood, which is crucial during chemotherapy (Chen et al., 2023). However, I also reassured Priya that rest is just as important and that she should listen to her body. Helping her find a sustainable balance between activity and rest was key to making sure she felt supported rather than pressured (Mast et al., 2024).

Priya's frustration with her taste changes was another moment that made me reflect on my role. She described a metallic taste that made it difficult for her to enjoy food, which is common among chemotherapy patients. I suggested simple but effective strategies, such as using plastic utensils, focusing on acidic or strong-flavoured foods, and staying hydrated (Sevryugin et al., 2021). I also encouraged her to approach this with a trial-and-error mindset, reassuring her that small changes might help her regain some control over her eating habits. This ties into my broader learning about patient empowerment – actively involving Priya in managing her own symptoms will give her more confidence and autonomy in her treatment journey (Zabernigg et al., 2010).

Reflecting on the pharmaceutical care model, I see how my role extends beyond dispensing medication – I am at the centre of symptom management, education, and patient empowerment. By working with Priya's GP and oncology team, I ensured she receives coordinated care that considers all aspects of her treatment. This case reaffirmed my belief that pharmacists can impact not just a patient's physical health but also their emotional and psychological well-being.

In conclusion, this case reinforced my understanding of the diverse and impactful role of community pharmacists in cancer care. Through education, evidence-based symptom management, and interprofessional collaboration, I can help enhance the quality of life for cancer patients like Priya. The values of patient empowerment, patient-centred care, and ethical decision-making are essential to this approach, ensuring that all patients receive comprehensive and compassionate support throughout their treatment journey.

Questions for reflection and discussion

Explore the key issues raised in the above scenario as you answer the following six questions:

1. How can pharmacists build trust with patients who are reluctant to share their diagnosis in a community pharmacy setting?

2. What strategies can be employed to improve patient awareness of the pharmacist's role in managing the side effects of cancer treatment?

3. How can pharmacists strengthen interprofessional communication to ensure comprehensive and coordinated care for patients like Priya?

4. How might the cumulative effect of chemotherapy influence the management of symptoms like fatigue and nausea over time?

5. In cases like Priya's, how can pharmacists support patients in making informed decisions about their treatment while managing expectations around symptom control?

6. What are the ethical considerations when discussing treatment side effects with a patient who is emotionally vulnerable?

Further reading

Hepler, C.D. and Strand, L.M. (1990) *Opportunities and responsibilities in pharmaceutical care. American Journal of Hospital Pharmacy*, 47: 533–543.

Macmillan Cancer Support (2022) *Understanding Chemotherapy*.

NHS England (2024a) *Aspirant Cancer Career and Education Development (ACCEND) Programme*. Available at: https://www.hee.nhs.uk/our-work/cancer-diagnostics/aspirant-cancer-career-education-development-programme/accend-framework (Accessed 30th September 2024).

NHS England (2024b) *How Pharmacies Can Help – NHS Services*. Available at: https://www.nhs.uk/nhs-services/pharmacies/how-pharmacies-can-help/ (Accessed 30th September 2024).

Royal Marsden (2024). *Online Manual of Clinical and Cancer Nursing Procedures*. 10th ed.

Further information

VALUES

Medicines safety focuses on ensuring that medications are prescribed, dispensed, and administered in a manner that maximises therapeutic benefit while minimising harm. This involves monitoring for drug interactions, preventing medication errors, and providing patient education on correct usage and potential side effects. The principles of medicines safety align with the World Health Organisation's global patient safety initiatives, which emphasise reducing preventable harm associated with medication use (World Health Organisation, 2022).

Patient autonomy refers to the patient's right to make informed decisions about their own healthcare, based on their individual values, beliefs, and preferences. It is a fundamental ethical principle in healthcare, ensuring that patients have control over their treatment choices. Pharmacists play a key role in supporting patient autonomy by providing evidence-based information and facilitating shared decision-making, particularly when discussing medication options and side effect management (Beauchamp and Childress, 2019).

Patient education involves providing patients with relevant information about their health, treatments, and procedures, enabling them to understand their condition and make informed decisions about their care. Effective patient education enhances health literacy, concordance with treatment plans, and overall health outcomes.

Patient empowerment refers to the process where patients gain control over their own health and healthcare decisions. It involves increasing patients' knowledge, skills, and confidence, thereby enabling them to actively manage their conditions. Empowerment is linked to improved health outcomes, particularly in managing long-term conditions, and supports a more collaborative relationship between patients and healthcare providers (Bravo et al., 2015).

Privacy in healthcare is an important aspect of protecting dignity and maintaining respect, the erosion of which can lead to a sense of violation of the self.

THEORIES

Behaviour change in health refers to the strategies and interventions used to support individuals in adopting healthier behaviours that contribute to better health outcomes. In the context of pharmacy, this includes encouraging adherence to medication regimens, promoting lifestyle modifications such as physical activity, and addressing barriers to behavioural change through motivational interviewing and personalised health advice. Behaviour change models, such as the COM-B framework (Capability, Opportunity, Motivation – Behaviour), provide structured approaches to understanding and influencing patient behaviour (Michie et al., 2011).

Concordance refers to a collaborative approach between healthcare professionals and patients in medication use, ensuring that treatment decisions align with the patient's preferences, beliefs, and lifestyle. Unlike adherence or compliance, which focuses on whether the patient follows prescribed instructions, concordance emphasises shared decision-making and mutual agreement. This approach improves patient engagement, satisfaction, and long-term treatment outcomes, particularly in chronic disease management (Royal Pharmaceutical Society, 2013).

Cumulative effects of chemotherapy refer to the increasing severity of side effects as treatment progresses due to the body's reduced ability to tolerate the repeated exposure to cytotoxic drugs. These effects often require adaptive management strategies, including pre-emptive interventions to maintain the patient's quality of life during treatment (Hertz et al., 2023).

Medicines optimisation is a person-centred approach to the safe and effective use of medicines, ensuring that patients receive the most appropriate medication for their condition while minimising risks and maximising benefits. This approach involves regular medication reviews, patient education, and interprofessional collaboration to tailor treatments to individual needs. Medicines optimisation aims to improve adherence, reduce polypharmacy-related complications, and enhance overall health outcomes (NHS England, 2023).

Non-pharmacological strategies are methods of managing symptoms without using medication. These strategies can include lifestyle interventions like diet modification, physical activity, relaxation techniques, and psychological counselling. Such approaches are often used to complement pharmacological treatments and help address various symptoms, including nausea and pain, in a holistic way.

Pharmaceutical care in oncology is the direct involvement of pharmacists in the treatment of cancer patients, aiming to optimise drug therapy, manage side effects, and improve quality of life. It includes personalised medication counselling, monitoring of therapeutic outcomes, and collaboration with other healthcare professionals to ensure effective treatment.

Symptom management is an approach aimed at minimising the physical and emotional discomfort caused by a condition or its treatment. It includes both pharmacological and non-pharmacological interventions to control symptoms such as pain, nausea, fatigue, and anxiety, thereby improving the patient's quality of life.

APPROACHES

Empathetic listening is the practice of being fully present and engaged while listening to a patient, attempting to understand their experiences and emotions from their perspective (Rogers, 1975). It is crucial for building a therapeutic relationship, fostering trust, and ensuring that patients feel heard and supported throughout their treatment.

Evidence-based pharmacotherapy involves applying the best available clinical evidence, patient preferences, and professional expertise to optimise medication use and improve health outcomes. Pharmacists use national and international guidelines, systematic reviews, and real-world data to ensure that treatments are safe, effective, and appropriate for individual patients. This approach reduces unnecessary medication use, minimises adverse effects, and supports personalised medicine (Sackett et al., 1996).

Health literacy refers to an individual's ability to access, understand, and use health information to make informed decisions about their care. A health literacy approach ensures that patients receive clear, accessible, and personalised information about their medications and treatment options. Low health literacy is associated with poor health outcomes, medication errors, and reduced adherence to treatment plans. Pharmacists play a crucial role in simplifying medical jargon, using teach-back techniques, and providing written materials to improve patient understanding (Nutbeam, 2008).

Patient-centred care involves tailoring healthcare interventions to align with individual patient needs, values, and preferences, emphasising respect for patient autonomy and involvement in decision-making. This approach ensures that the patient remains at the core of all healthcare processes and decisions. It fosters trust and empowers patients to be active participants in managing their health, which can significantly enhance their well-being and quality of care.

Patient engagement involves actively involving patients in their own healthcare, encouraging them to take part in decision-making processes, and educating them about their health conditions and treatment options. Engaged patients tend to experience better outcomes, as they are more likely to follow treatment plans and make informed decisions about their health (Hickmann et al., 2022).

Shared decision-making focuses on including patients in all decisions about their own lives so that their voices are heard and their individual preferences understood and fully represented in any decision-making process which takes place.

Symptom management refers to the use of various interventions to alleviate symptoms associated with a disease or its treatment. It may involve a combination of pharmacological measures (e.g., pain relievers, antiemetics) and non-pharmacological approaches (e.g., dietary changes, exercise) to improve a patient's quality of life during treatment.

MODELS

Integrated care model focuses on collaboration among various healthcare professionals, including GPs, oncologists, pharmacists, and dietitians, to provide comprehensive and coordinated care. This model aims to reduce fragmentation of services, improve continuity of care, and address complex patient needs more effectively. The approach has been shown to improve patient outcomes by enhancing the integration between primary, secondary, and community healthcare services, ensuring patients receive cohesive support across different stages of their care journey (Baxter et al., 2018).

Pharmaceutical care model emphasises the responsible provision of drug therapy to achieve specific patient outcomes that enhance quality of life. It involves the pharmacist collaborating closely with both the patient and other healthcare providers to optimise medication use, manage side effects, and ensure that all medication-related needs are addressed (Hepler and Grainger-Rousseau, 1995). This model is crucial in long-term condition management, where ongoing adjustments in therapy may be necessary to manage symptoms and side effects effectively (Alves da Costa et al., 2019).

The biopsychosocial model, proposed by Engel (1977), acknowledges that health and illness are influenced by a combination of biological (e.g., disease pathology), psychological (such as emotional well-being and stress), and social (e.g., relationships and support networks) factors. In pharmacy practice, this model highlights the need for a holistic approach to patient care, addressing not only pharmacological treatments but also psychological support and lifestyle modifications. For cancer patients like Priya, recognising the interaction between physical symptoms, emotional distress, and social support is key to improving overall well-being (Borrell-Carrió et al., 2004).

References

Alves da Costa, F., Foppe van Mil, J.W. and Alvarez-Risco, A. (2019) *The Pharmacist Guide to Implementing Pharmaceutical Care*. Springer International Publishing.

Baxter, S., Johnson, M., Chambers, D., Sutton, A., Goyder, E. and Booth, A. (2018) The effects of integrated care: A systematic review of UK and international evidence. *BMC Health Services Research*, 18, 350.

Beauchamp, T.L. and Childress, J.F. (2019) *Principles of Biomedical Ethics*. 8th edn. Oxford: Oxford University Press.

Borrell-Carrió, F., Suchman, A.L. and Epstein, R.M. (2004) The biopsychosocial model 25 years later: Principles, practice, and scientific inquiry. *Annals of Family Medicine*, 2(6), 576–582.

Bravo, P., Edwards, A., Barr, P.J., Scholl, I., Elwyn, G., McAllister, M. and the Cochrane Healthcare Quality Research Group, C U (2015) Conceptualising patient empowerment: A mixed methods study. *BMC Health Services Research*, 15, 252.

Chen, X., Li, J., Chen, C., Zhang, Y., Zhang, S., Zhang, Y., Zhou, L. and Hu, X. (2023) Effects of exercise interventions on cancer-related fatigue and quality of life among cancer patients: A meta-analysis. *BMC Nursing*, 22, 200.

Engel, G.L. (1977) The need for a new medical model: A challenge for biomedicine. *Science*, 196(4286), 129–136.

Gupta, K., Walton, R. and Kataria, S. (2020) Chemotherapy-induced nausea and vomiting: Pathogenesis, recommendations, and new trends. *Cancer Treatment and Research Communications*, 26, 100278.

Hepler, C.D. and Grainger-Rousseau, T-J. (1995) Pharmaceutical care versus traditional drug treatment: Is there a difference? *Drugs*, 49, 1–10.

Hertz, D.L., Lustberg, M.B. and Sonis, S. (2023) Evolution of predictive risk factor analysis for chemotherapy-related toxicity. *Supportive Care in Cancer*, 31, 601.

Hickmann, E., Richter, P. and Schlieter, H. (2022) All together now – patient engagement, patient empowerment, and associated terms in personal healthcare. *BMC Health Services Research*, 22, 1116.

Mast, I.H., Bongers, C.C.W.G., Gootjes, E.C., de Wilt, J.H.W., Hopman, M.T.E. and Buffart, L.M. (2024) Potential mechanisms underlying the effect of walking exercise on cancer-related fatigue in cancer survivors. *Journal of Cancer Survivorship*, 1–12. https://doi.org/10.1007/s11764-024-01537-y

McCormack, B., McCance, T., Bulley, C., Brown, D., McMillan, A. and Martin, S. (2021) *Fundamentals of Person-Centred Healthcare Practice*. Wiley.

Michie, S., van Stralen, M.M. and West, R. (2011) The behaviour change wheel: A new method for characterising and designing behaviour change interventions. *Implementation Science*, 6, 42.

NHS England (2023) *Medicines Optimisation: Helping Patients to Make the Most of Medicines*. Available at: https://www.england.nhs.uk/medicines-optimisation/ (Accessed 17th February 2025).

Nutbeam, D. (2008) The evolving concept of health literacy. *Social Science & Medicine*, 67(12), 2072–2078.

Rogers, C.R. (1975) Empathic: An unappreciated way of being. *The Counselling Psychologist*, 5, 2–10.

Royal Pharmaceutical Society (2013) *Medicines Adherence: Involving Patients in Decisions about Medicines and Supporting Adherence* [Online]. Available at: https://www.nice.org.uk/guidance/cg76/resources/medicines-adherence-pdf-975631782085 (Accessed 17th February 2025).

Sackett, D.L., Rosenberg, W.M., Gray, J.A., Haynes, R.B. and Richardson, W.S. (1996) Evidence-based medicine: What it is and what it isn't. *BMJ*, 312(7023), 71–72.

Sevryugin, O., Kasvis, P., Vigano, M. and Vigano, A. (2021) Taste and smell disturbances in cancer patients: A scoping review of available treatments. *Supportive Care in Cancer*, 29, 49–66.

World Health Organization (WHO) (2022) *Medication without Harm – WHO Global Patient Safety Challenge on Medication Safety*. Available at: https://www.who.int/initiatives/medication-without-harm (Accessed 17th February 2025).

Zabernigg, A., Gamper, E-M., Giesinger, J.M., Rumpold, G., Kemmler, G., Gattringer, K., Sperner-Unterweger, B. and Holzner, B. (2010) Taste alterations in cancer patients receiving chemotherapy: A neglected side effect? *The Oncologist*, 15, 913–920.

Case study 13
Becky: moving forward

Paul Linsley

Becky's referral

I first met Becky after she had been diagnosed with triple-negative breast cancer. Following surgery and treatment, she had experienced several years of active and fulfilling life. However, eight years later, Becky began feeling fatigued and lost her appetite. Further tests revealed that her cancer had returned, spreading to the lymph nodes in her armpits. Despite undergoing chemotherapy, and chemoradiotherapy, the cancer continued to progress, spreading to other parts of her body. Becky has now been given six months to a year to live.

APPROACH: chemotherapy

APPROACH: chemoradiotherapy

Meeting Becky again

As a community nurse, I have cared for many individuals at various stages of their cancer journey. No two experiences are the same. Some patients struggle to reconcile their diagnosis with their sense of self, while others find meaning in it. For couples, cancer can place unique strains on relationships, sometimes bringing them closer together and at other times creating distance. Understanding the individuality of each patient is crucial to providing compassionate and effective care.

VALUE: valuing people

Knowing the complexity of Becky's situation, I schedule a double appointment for our first visit, to ensure she has time to share as much as she wants to. Given that Becky's cancer has now spread to her lungs, I need to assess her breathing and overall well-being.

APPROACH: clinical decision-making

Becky greets me at the front door, her smile warm but weary. Introducing myself, I follow her into the living room, where she gestures for me to take a seat opposite her. She appears frail, her clothes hanging loosely on her frame. I

APPROACH: "Hello, my name is..." campaign

DOI: 10.4324/9781003651758-13

notice a slight tremor in her hand as she holds a glass of water. This may be a side effect of medication or an indication of anxiety, something I plan to explore as our conversation progresses.

'I guess you have lots of questions,' Becky said, shifting in her seat.

I lean forward slightly, adopting an open posture. 'As this is my first visit, I am happy to be led by you. What would you like to talk about? I will need to assess your breathing at some point, but I'm happy to explore anything else first.'

She takes a moment before answering. 'I don't know where to start. It's all been a bit of a whirlwind since I left hospital. Friends keep dropping by, keeping me busy, as if they're afraid of leaving me alone. Everyone's determined to get me out of the house.'

She sighs, her shoulders slumping slightly. 'I know they mean well, but I can't help feeling like I'm being smothered. They're treating me like I'm fragile, like I might break at any moment. I'm still me, you know? I don't want to be seen only as someone who is sick. I want to feel normal again, even if just for a little while.'

She pauses. 'Honestly, I don't feel much different than when I was well. I'm still eating, still exercising. I was – am – a runner. I still go out most nights.'

'It's great that you can still do something that you love and enjoy,' I reply.

She visibly relaxes. 'I'm determined to make the most of the time I have left.'

As she speaks, I listen, letting her take the lead. My role is not just to assess her physical health but to support her in telling her story. So much of palliative care is about giving patients space to express their fears, hopes, and realities. Knowing when to step in and when to step back is a delicate balance.

'I always knew the cancer would return,' Becky admits suddenly. 'It never really left; it was always living rent-free in my head.' She sighs deeply, 'I do worry, but I try to stay positive.'

VALUE: self-determination

She hesitates before continuing, her gaze dropping to her hands. 'My family is my biggest concern. My husband is supportive, but I can tell he's struggling.' Her brow furrows as she reflects. 'He tries to be strong for me, but I see the toll it's taking on him. He's always worried about what I need, and I can feel the weight of that responsibility on his shoulders. Sometimes I wish he'd just let himself feel - let himself be angry or sad instead of putting on a brave face.'

Becky pauses, her fingers fidgeting with the hem of her sweater. 'And then there's my daughter, Lucy. She's spending so much time with me - more than is normal for a teenager. I guess that's natural, but I even find it hard to go to the bathroom alone,' she laughs lightly, though the humour does not quite reach her eyes. 'I feel guilty for needing her so much. I want her to have her own life, to hang out with friends, to do all the things teenagers should be doing. But here I am, making her my priority, and I can see it's weighing on her. She shouldn't have to take care of me; it should be the other way around.'

VALUE: understanding

Her expression quickly turns serious as she leans forward, 'It's my mum I worry about most. She's not coping. She cries every time she visits, and I try to reassure her, to tell them all that I'm managing, but it's exhausting.' Becky's eyes glisten with unshed tears; a mixture of love and concern for her mother is evident in her gaze. 'I feel like I have to put on this brave front for them, but sometimes I just want to scream. It's hard to balance my own fears with their expectations. I don't want them to suffer because of me.'

Hearing Becky's pain

She takes a sip of water, her voice softer now, almost a whisper, 'The hardest part of dying is meeting other people's expectations. It's draining.' A heavy silence fills the room as her words hang in the air, a poignant reflection of the emotional burden she carries.

She looks at me directly, her eyes searching for understanding. 'I want to be remembered for three things: that I was a good wife, a good mother, and a good person.' Each word feels weighted, a declaration of her identity that she fears might slip away with her illness.

VALUE: compassion and empathy

Then, without warning, she breaks into uncontrollable crying. I sit in silence, allowing her space to grieve and release the emotions she has been holding back for her family's sake. It is a powerful moment, watching her vulnerability surface. Through her tears, she says, 'I don't want to die.'

APPROACH: emotional support

Many clinicians feel the need to respond, to offer words of comfort, but in these moments, the best response is often the simplest. 'This is clearly a distressing time for you,' I say gently, acknowledging her reality without diminishing her emotions.

APPROACH: emotional support

As her cry echoes in the room, I feel the profound sadness that accompanies her journey – the weight of expectations, the fear of leaving her loved ones, and the pain of feeling like a burden. I am careful to manage my own emotions in response to Becky's disclosure, while acknowledging the distress that she is under.

APPROACH: emotional intelligence

After several minutes, Becky takes a deep breath, wiping away her tears with the back of her hand. 'I'm sorry,' she says, her voice shaky. 'Sometimes it just catches me off guard, and I don't know how to hold it all in anymore.'

APPROACH: emotional support

'There's no need to apologise,' I reassure her gently. 'This is your space to feel however you need and want to feel.'

VALUES: compassion and empathy and building trust

Becky nods, her expression shifting as she rallies herself. 'I've been trying to remind myself to be positive, to focus on the good moments. I don't want to sit around waiting for the end. I want to make memories. I want to live.' Her determination is palpable, a flicker of strength in the middle of deep vulnerability.

VALUE: respect for autonomy

Still Becky

We sit together for a moment longer, the weight of her emotions still lingering in the air. I admire her resilience and her desire to find meaning within such uncertainty. It is a delicate balance – navigating the pain of her journey while also embracing the moments that bring her joy.

MODEL: The Dual Process Model of Coping with Bereavement

She shows me a list she has made – things she wants to do while she still has enough energy. Some are grand plans, like a family trip to the Lake District, a place she has always loved. Others are simple but meaningful – afternoon tea with her closest friends, a picnic with her daughter in their favourite park, or even just watching the sunrise with her husband while wrapped in a warm blanket.

'My body might be failing, but I'm still here,' she says. 'And I want to make sure that the people I love remember me not as someone who was sick, but as someone who lived.'

APPROACH: holistic approach

She has taken up journaling and writing letters to her daughter and husband, filled with memories, advice, and love. 'I want Lucy to have something to hold onto,' she explains, 'I want her to know how much she was loved.'

Becky's energy is contagious, and despite the weight of her prognosis, there is light in her eyes when she speaks of the things she is planning. 'I refuse to let cancer steal what time I have left,' she says with a smile, 'I'm still Becky. I'm still me.'

A shift in focus

Becky's transition from curative to palliative care is not just a clinical process but an emotional and psychological journey, I think to myself. The shift in focus, from fighting the disease to maximising quality of life – can be challenging. Many patients feel powerless in this transition.

MODEL: The Four Domains Model

Empowering them to take an active role in their care can help them manage uncertainty and maintain resilience.

For the rest of the visit, I conduct the necessary assessments while continuing our conversation about her family and the support she is receiving. As Becky is transitioning from curative to palliative care, she is also transitioning from fighting cancer to finding peace in the time she has left. My role is to support her in that transition, not just medically but emotionally, helping her to tell her story on her own terms.

As I leave, I reflect on our conversation. Every interaction with a patient is different, requiring adaptability, sensitivity, and presence. Becky's story is hers to tell, and I am here to listen, validate, and support her as she navigates this final chapter of her life.

Reflection

Reflecting on my visit with Becky, I found myself contemplating the profound transition that patients with terminal illnesses experience as they move from curative to palliative care. This shift is not just a change in treatment goals; it represents a deeply emotional journey for patients, their families, and healthcare professionals alike. It requires a delicate balance between resilience and acceptance, a process that can be incredibly challenging.

One of the most striking aspects of this transition is the mental and emotional adjustment it demands. Many patients have been conditioned to fight their illness at all costs, making it difficult to reframe their perspective when curative treatment is no longer an option (Kitta et al., 2021). Understanding when a patient is ready to shift focus to palliative care can profoundly impact their experience and overall well-being (Hov et al., 2020). Often, this awareness emerges when the burdens of aggressive treatment become overwhelming or when the realisation sets in that their prognosis is no longer favourable. My role as a nurse is to approach this transition with sensitivity, allowing patients to guide the conversation based on their emotional and physical readiness. By being attuned to their cues, I can provide the necessary support without rushing or forcing the process.

Preparation is equally vital. I have learned that equipping both patients and their families with knowledge and resources helps them navigate the palliative approach with more confidence. Anticipating the questions and concerns that may arise allows me to provide clear, compassionate explanations about what palliative care truly means. It is essential to convey that palliative care is not about giving up – it is about living well with the time that remains. By framing it in this way, patients and families can be empowered to engage actively in decision-making and feel more in control.

Effective communication stands out as the most critical factor in this process. Establishing open, honest conversations fosters trust between patients, families, and healthcare providers. I strive to create a safe space where patients feel comfortable expressing their fears, hopes, and desires. Actively listening to their concerns allows me to address their emotional needs while providing the medical information they require. During my visit with Becky, the emotional weight of her diagnosis was evident. Validating her feelings and encouraging her to share her story significantly enhanced her experience of care.

I was grateful for the double appointment I had scheduled. These conversations should never feel rushed; patients with terminal illness often fluctuate between hopefulness and realism (Gardiner et al., 2015). Becky shared deeply personal thoughts and fears, reminding me of the unique and profound nature of the nurse-patient relationship. I recognise that patients often confide in healthcare professionals in ways they may not be with their families, and I deeply respect the trust they place in me.

Another vital lesson from my visit was recognising the different types of conversations we engage in as nurses. Practical discussions about symptom management must coexist with emotional conversations that offer empathy and understanding, as well as social conversations that help patients maintain a sense of normality. Being mindful of the type of conversation taking place allows me to tailor my approach accordingly. By allowing Becky to take the lead, I was able to support her in a way that was truly meaningful.

Recognising different conversation phases, such as introduction, assessment, intervention, and closure, has helped me refine my communication strategies. Understanding the structure of our conversations allows me to enhance my skills, ultimately improving patient care and outcomes. One of the most valuable lessons I have learned is that the patient is always the best author of their own story. Each patient's journey is unique, and our conversations should honour their individual experiences. By fostering trust, ensuring transparency, and providing both emotional and clinical support, I can help patients like Becky find peace and purpose in the time they have left.

At its core, I believe the nurse-patient relationship is underpinned by trust. When I enter this relationship, I commit to respecting my patients' autonomy, maintaining their confidentiality, explaining treatment options, obtaining informed consent, providing the highest standard of care, and ensuring that I do not abandon them (Allande-Cussó et al., 2021). However, I find that the essential elements of clinical encounters, such as building relationships, opening discussions, gathering information, understanding perspectives, sharing information, reaching agreements, and providing closure, often fail to capture the depth of this connection and the complexity of the work undertaken. Patients frequently share secrets, worries, and fears with me that they have not yet disclosed to their loved ones, and I hold this trust with the utmost care.

When discussing treatment and care, I continuously assess the patient's emotional state, readiness, and understanding, tailoring my conversation accordingly. Patients like Becky frequently express anxiety, fear, sadness, and anger, so recognising these emotions is essential to effective communication. I often employ a three-stage model: recognising emotions through active listening, exploring emotions by acknowledging and validating them, and managing distress through empathetic information provision and referrals (Stiefel et al., 2024). This attentiveness builds trust and reassures patients that they are truly being heard.

Facilitating a supportive narrative around palliative care is something I believe is crucial in my role as a nurse. I often encounter patients who fear this stage of their journey, associating it with loss, despair, and the end of hope. However, I have come to understand that when palliative care is framed positively, it represents much more than that – it is about living well for as long as possible. It emphasises comfort, dignity, and maintaining a sense of control during a time that can feel overwhelmingly uncertain.

As I work with patients and families, such as Becky, I remind myself that my approach can significantly influence their experience during this transition. I am committed to providing them with the tools and support they need to feel secure and cared for, ensuring they know that they have a partner in this journey. Ultimately, I hope that by fostering a positive understanding of palliative care, I can help alleviate some of the fears associated with it and promote a sense of peace and acceptance for my patients and their families.

While many nurses find working with cancer patients rewarding, it can also be emotionally taxing. I have seen how clinicians sometimes fear getting too close to patients, erecting barriers to shield themselves from emotional fatigue. It is common to experience anxiety, sadness, and frustration when listening to patients' stories. When Becky shared memories of her daughter Lucy, I felt a surge of emotion, reminded of my own experience of losing my mother to cancer as a teenager. Though I chose not to disclose this personal history, it reinforced the emotional demands of my work and the importance of self-awareness in nursing practice. Recognising how my own experiences might influence my conversations with patients is a critical part of providing empathetic and professional care.

Nursing is more than providing medical care. It is about being present, listening deeply, and affirming the humanity of the individuals with whom we work. It is about ensuring patients feel seen, heard, and valued. By prioritising open communication and patient-centred care, I can help ease the transition from curative to palliative treatment and improve the quality of life for those facing terminal illnesses. My experience with Becky reinforced the importance of these principles and reminded me why I chose to be a nurse in the first place: to provide care that is not only clinically sound but also deeply compassionate and meaningful.

Two guiding principles shape my clinical practice: 'It's not until the person knows you care that they care about what you know,' and 'You're only as good as your last conversation.' These reminders push me to approach every interaction with empathy, intention, and an unwavering commitment to making a difference in patients' lives.

Questions for reflection and discussion

Explore the key issues raised in the above scenario as you answer the following six questions:

1. How do you typically prepare yourself mentally and emotionally before initiating difficult conversations with patients and their families?

2. What specific topics do you find most challenging to discuss with patients, and how do you navigate these discomforts to ensure that patient care is not compromised?

3. In what ways do your feelings of discomfort or avoidance during some conversations influence the quality of care and support you provide to your patients?

4. When faced with a patient's sudden emotional shift, what immediate steps would you take to address their needs while maintaining a supportive and compassionate environment?

5. How do the core values of care and compassion manifest in your daily interactions with patients, especially during emotionally charged conversations?

6. Can you identify a specific instance where you encountered a challenging emotion in your professional role? What strategies did you use to work through it, and what insights did you gain from that experience?

Further reading

Davis, M. P. and LeGrand, S. B. (2020) Addressing the emotional distress of patients with cancer: A review of literature and recommendations. *Palliative Medicine*, 34(9): 1123–1132.

Dean, M. and Street, R.L. (2014) A 3-stage model of patient-centered communication for addressing cancer patients' emotional distress. *Patient Education and Counselling*, 94(2): 143–148.

Harris, R. J. and Egan, M. (2021) The role of communication in cancer care: Improving patient outcomes through better conversations. *Supportive Care in Cancer*, 29(5): 2053–2060.

Pereira, J. A. and Horneber, M. (2020) Transitioning from curative to palliative care: Challenges and recommendations. *Journal of Cancer Research and Clinical Oncology*, 146(2): 513–523.

Rosenberg, J. and Zoloth, L. (2022) Patient-centered communication in oncology: Moving beyond treatment to embrace the emotional journey. *Oncology Nursing Forum*, 49(1): 45–53.

Further information

VALUES

Building trust is a fundamental value in healthcare. It ensures that patients feel safe, respected, and confident in the care they receive. Trust is built through honesty, reliability, competence, and compassionate communication.

Caring involves empathy, compassion, and a commitment to the well-being of others, ensuring that patients receive not only medical treatment but also emotional and psychological support.

Compassion and empathy involve understanding a patient's emotions and experiences and offering kindness and emotional support.

Respect for autonomy is honouring the patient's wishes regarding their care preferences and end-of-life decisions.

Self-determination is a core value in nursing and healthcare and emphasises individuals' right to make free choices without external compulsion. However, the concept is not without challenges. In adult protection, practitioners struggle to balance empowerment and protection, rights, and risks.

Understanding involves having a sympathetic awareness of another person's thoughts, feelings, and experiences and is central to providing person-centred care, as well as to providing approaches which help to avoid stress and distress for patients of all backgrounds and abilities.

Valuing people regardless of our differences in background, belief, culture, and outlook is fundamental to respectful healthcare delivery. Person-centred interactions that value, acknowledge, and validate the individual make a huge contribution to an individual's well-being.

APPROACHES

Active listening is a communication technique that enhances mutual understanding and improves relationships. It involves fully focusing on the speaker, providing feedback, and responding empathetically. By creating a safe and a stimulating environment, active listening encourages free expression of thoughts and feelings.

Chemotherapy is a cancer treatment that utilises one or more anti-cancer drugs to destroy rapidly dividing cells. While effective against cancer, chemotherapy can cause various side effects due to its impact on normal rapidly dividing cells, including fatigue, nausea, hair loss, and increased infection risk.

Chemoradiotherapy (CRT) combines chemotherapy and radiotherapy to treat locally advanced solid tumours.

Clinical decision-making (CDM) is a complex process involving information processing, evidence evaluation, and knowledge application to select appropriate interventions for high-quality patient care. It encompasses both intuitive and analytical thinking patterns. Challenges to CDM include the expanding clinical knowledge base, data timeliness, and care complexity.

Clinical observation is a fundamental skill for nurses, encompassing initial patient assessment and long-term monitoring and assessment of the person in undertaking tasks within their environment.

Emotional intelligence (EI) is the ability to recognise, understand, and manage emotions in oneself and others. It encompasses skills such as identifying and discriminating among emotions and using emotional information to guide thinking and actions. Some researchers suggest that EI can be learned and strengthened, while others argue it is an innate characteristic.

Emotional support Key elements of emotional support include warmth, kindness, deep listening, and fostering social connections during treatment.

'Hello, my name is…' campaign, initiated by Dr Kate Granger (2016), encourages healthcare professionals to introduce themselves to patients, promoting compassionate care.

Holistic Approach is considering not only physical health but also emotional, social, spiritual, and psychological well-being of the person.

Patient empowerment is a concept that promotes autonomous self-regulation and maximises an individual's potential for health and wellness. It involves patients gaining knowledge, skills, and attitudes to actively participate in their healthcare decisions and improve their quality of life.

Person-centred care is an approach to healthcare that respects and responds to the unique needs, preferences, and values of individuals. It prioritises the person rather than just their illness, ensuring that care is tailored to their personal circumstances, beliefs, and goals.

Supportive communication plays a crucial role in cancer patient care, enhancing psychological adjustment and coping abilities. Effective clinician-patient communication can be improved through formal supportive care screening and discussion processes, which help patients reflect on their needs and initiate conversations. Nurses should develop interpersonal communication skills to recognise nonverbal cues and respond appropriately to patients' concerns.

Therapeutic communication is a crucial aspect of nursing care, involving interpersonal interaction between nurses and patients to address health issues. It is fundamental to establishing effective nurse-client relationships and is considered key to the therapeutic process. The approach encompasses various techniques, including exploration, affirmation, and reframing, aimed at facilitating patient understanding and promoting positive change.

MODELS

The **Dual Process Model** of coping with bereavement, developed by Margaret Stroebe and Henk Schut (1999), explains how individuals navigate grief by oscillating between two types of coping processes: loss-oriented and restoration-oriented coping. This model acknowledges that grief is not a linear process but involves dynamic movement between confronting and avoiding loss.

The **Four Domains Model** of Palliative Care (National Consensus Project for Quality Palliative Care, 2018) provides a framework for addressing the comprehensive needs of patients with serious illnesses. It ensures that care goes beyond physical symptoms to include psychological, social, and spiritual well-being. This model is widely used in palliative and end-of-life care to guide holistic, person-centred support.

References

Allande-Cussó, R., Rodríguez-Mañas, L. and Lázaro, J. (2021) Ethical dilemmas in the treatment of patients with advanced illness: A review of the literature. *Journal of Medical Ethics*, 47(4): 239–246. https://doi.org/10.1136/medethics-2020-106506

Gardiner, C., Ingleton, C., Gott, M. and Ryan, T. (2015) Exploring the transition from curative care to palliative care: A systematic review of the literature. *BMJ Supportive and Palliative Care*, 5(4): 335–342. ISSN 2045-435X.

Granger, K. (2016) "Hello, my name is…" and its impact on the patient experience: A conversation with Dr Kate Granger. *BMJ Quality & Safety*, 25(3): 181–184. doi: 10.1136/bmjqs-2015-004486.

Hov, L., Synnes, O. and Aarseth, G. (2020) Negotiating the turning point in the transition from curative to palliative treatment: A linguistic analysis of medical records of dying patients. *BMC Palliative Care*, 19, 91. https://doi.org/10.1186/s12904-020-00602-4

Kitta, A., Hagin, A., Unseld, M., Adamidis, F., Diendorfer, T., Masel, E. K. and Kirchheiner, K. (2021) The silent transition from curative to palliative treatment: A qualitative study about cancer patients' perceptions of end-of-life discussions with oncologists. *Supportive Care in Cancer: Official Journal of the Multinational Association of Supportive Care in Cancer*, 29(5): 2405–2413. https://doi.org/10.1007/s00520-020-05750-0

National Consensus Project for Quality Palliative Care. (2018) *Clinical Practice Guidelines for Quality Palliative Care*, 4th edition. National Coalition for Hospice and Palliative Care. Retrieved from https://www.nationalcoalitionhpc.org [Last Accessed: 20.02.25]

Stiefel, F., Bourquin, C., Salmon, P., Achtari Jeanneret, L., Dauchy, S., Ernstmann, N., Grassi, L., Libert, Y., Vitinius, F., Santini, D. and Ripamonti, C.I.; ESMO (2024) Guidelines Committee: Communication and Support of Patients and Caregivers in Chronic Cancer Care: ESMO Clinical Practice Guideline. *ESMO Open*, 9(7): 103496. doi: 10.1016/j.esmoop.2024.103496. Epub 2024 Jun 18. PMID: 39089769; PMCID: PMC11360426.

Stroebe, M. and Schut, H. (1999) The Dual Process Model of Coping with Bereavement: Rationale and Description. *Death Studies*, 23(3): 197–224. https://doi.org/10.1080/074811899201046

Case study 14
Will: it is hard to say much

Chrysi Leliopoulou

Will's background

As community cancer nurses, we often work with individuals who do not always want to engage in discussions
about their treatment and prognosis. Therefore, community nurses may find themselves needing to tease out
issues and initiate difficult conversations with patients who
have a cancer diagnosis. Discussing treatment options and
end-of-life care can be uncomfortable, and many patients
and their families may be apprehensive and overwhelmed
by their situation, being far from ready to discuss strong
emotions such as anger, fear, and frustration. Sometimes,
patients may experience isolation and loneliness as they
struggle to communicate their hopelessness and sadness.
Supporting patients to connect with their own feelings
often requires high levels of awareness and advanced communication skills to support the untangling of an emotional
mayhem and psychological distress.

THEORY: end-of-life care

THEORY: hopelessness

APPROACH: empathy

After visiting Will and his wife Mary a fortnight ago, a
colleague has requested a follow-up visit from the team. I
offer to visit to find out how they are coping with Will's terminal diagnosis. My colleague has noted that over the past
few months, Will has reported having episodes of choking
and sputtering after most of his meals. Initially, these
episodes were brief and infrequent, but over time, they
became more regular and longer lasting. Mary had urged
Will to see a doctor, but Will did not think his symptoms
were serious and was focused on his business. He thought
Mary was over-concerned and fussed over him, which he
found a little irritating. Eventually, he agreed to see a doctor,
who initially misdiagnosed him with thrush in his throat.

THEORY: disease progression

APPROACH: misdiagnosis and mistreatment

The doctor prescribed treatment for Will for a few weeks, but
his symptoms got worse and persistent, with his coughing
and choking becoming more frequent and severe. He also

DOI: 10.4324/9781003651758-14

developed a hoarse voice and eventually was referred for tests for pneumonia and tuberculosis. Will had been slightly concerned as his symptoms worsened, but was confident that the doctors knew what they were doing.

THEORY: closed awareness

For some time, Mary had been hearing Will get up during the night because of coughing and choking on his own saliva. Looking back on these incidents, Mary now realises that this is not just a simple cough, and wishes she had pressed Will more to go back to the GP. One of the reasons for my visit, it is that Mary has reported being upset and tearful after Will's last hospital appointment, at which they were told that his cancer is terminal.

Meeting Will and Mary

When I enter the flat, Mary greets me with a smile, but she quickly looks away as she says, 'Hello.' Will is silent, completely absorbed or lost in thought, staring at the television.

I smile and say, 'Hello,' but Will does not respond; his expression is blank, and I wonder if he even notices I am here. I rub my hands together unnoticed, and then his eyes shift and meet mine. His gaze is tired, exhausted, and somehow troubled.

THEORY: managing strong emotions

'Hello! How are you today, Will?' I ask. He leans back against the sofa cushions, looks at me, and reluctantly replies, 'Okay, I guess.' His expression makes me briefly smile at him as I sit on the chair opposite him, and we start talking about the weather. We agree it is miserable this morning, windy, and rainy.

MODEL: communication skills

I know from the case notes that Will is a 77-year-old retired greengrocer who lives with his wife Mary, and their youngest son. His other two children live abroad. Will has been diagnosed with oesophageal cancer and has just started attending the outpatient clinic at his local hospital for fortnightly palliative chemotherapy treatment.

Will is keen to have dinner with his wife to keep things normal, but recently he has been struggling to keep any food or drink is difficult to swallow because of the cough and choking, so sitting at the table at meals is becoming a struggle for him. He currently only manages sips of water and liquidised food. In the past two weeks, his voice has also changed and become hoarser and croakier. He is tired, which makes it hard to hold a conversation, so he has become quieter and more withdrawn. Mary feels that he is fading away, and the whole family is finding Will's diagnosis difficult.

THEORY: suspected awareness

MODEL: coping strategies

Mary feels it was Will's unwillingness to follow-up on his symptoms that took away his chance of timely treatment. Mary has also had an argument with their oldest daughter, who is upset about her dad's diagnosis and blames her mother for not making him go to the doctors' quicker. Her distress has made things worse for Mary and Will.

MODEL: stages of grief

THEORY: coping

I am concerned about the emotional burden Mary is carrying and enquire further, 'How are you getting on?'

Mary responds, 'I'm fine, really. It's the family that has been upsetting me.'

Mary appears exhausted. I wonder how the stress is affecting her and whether she is experiencing a sense of helplessness. Relatives often struggle with feelings of helplessness, on top of being fearful about their loved one's condition. I mirror her words to explore this further, asking: 'How has the family been upsetting you?'.

THEORY: despondency

APPROACH: mirroring

'I can't bear it,' she says.

'What is it that you can't bear?' I think I understand what she means, but I ask anyway to provide Mary with the opportunity to say more. Mary is quiet, not immediately responding. I offer to make some tea for us all. Mary gets up, and I follow her into the kitchen. Will remains quiet, not reacting to us moving into the kitchen. He continues watching the television. I feel quite upset having observed the silence between the two of them.

APPROACH: empathy

I reach out to the tap to fill the kettle when Mary asks, 'What's going on with Will? Will he get better?' I wait for a few moments, and then, looking at the kettle as it begins to warm up, I meet her eyes and say, 'What did the doctors say to you when you saw them last?'

I know Mary is not ready to accept the bad news, so I pause and pull out the kitchen chair to sit down, saying, 'I know the doctors have spoken with you and Will about the next steps. What did you understand from what they said last week? How did the kids react to the news?' I can sense Mary knows but does not want to accept the news.

Is he really dying?

APPROACH: managing strong emotions

'Is he really dying?' She asks. I calmly reply 'Yes' and apart from the boiling kettle, the room is quiet.

APPROACH: empathy

VALUE: truth-telling

THEORY: closed awareness

It is important to acknowledge silences but also respond calmly. 'I can see you're feeling uncertain. It's okay to feel that way. Mary, I want to understand what's making you ask this now.' Mary, with a trembling voice, responds, 'I didn't realise it was this serious. I never suspected. He was always so strong and healthy, working at the shop all the time. What happened?'

THEORY: hopelessness

After a pause, she continues, 'He didn't go to the doctor early enough. I told him so many times, but he wouldn't listen. He just kept working at the shop, and now you say he is dying.'

As the rain begins to fall again, we hear the droplets tapping on the glass windows. Through the slightly open door, we can see Will, absent-mindedly watching the news on the television.

THEORY: despondency

'Have you talked to Will about how you're feeling?' I ask. Mary shakes her head and replies through gritted teeth, 'He doesn't talk.' I can feel the depth of her pain as she clenches her fist and holds her arm against her stomach.

APPROACH: mirroring

'I'm sorry, Mary. This must be incredibly hard for you. How can I help you and the family?' Her face grimaces, and I feel sad for her. Giving permission to feel unsure, angry, and upset is important when breaking bad news, so I say, 'I can see you are unsure. It is okay to be unsure, Mary. But I'd really like to find out what is making you so upset and angry about the situation now?'

Mary's voice breaks a bit as she replies: 'I feel he doesn't care about me.'

I ask, 'Have you spoken to Will about how you feel?'

Mary nods and, through clenched teeth, says, 'He doesn't want to talk.'

'I am sorry,' I say, 'This must be hard for you, Mary. How does that make you feel?'

After a pause, she replies: 'Empty, frustrated.'

I say, 'I'm really sorry to hear that Mary, do you want me to speak with Will for you?'

Is she okay?

Leaving Mary in the kitchen, I walk back into the lounge with my cup of tea and sit across from Will, saying, 'How have you been keeping, Will?'

Will looks at me and replies, 'I don't know. I'm a bit worried about Mary and the kids. They've been arguing a lot lately, and they don't get on well.'

I feel a bit uneasy but ask, 'How do you mean?'

Will continues, 'I feel like I need to be a bit more open with Mary and make things right for her, but I don't know how.'

I sense Will is fearful of upsetting Mary and the kids further and feels under a lot of stress. So, I say, 'How about I talk to Mary about this, is that okay?' I take a sip of my tea just as Mary walks back into the room. The rain has stopped, and as I sit there on the sofa, I say, 'I'll make another round of tea. Mary, why don't you sit here with Will and tell him what you asked me earlier in the kitchen, is that okay? I'll join you in a moment or two.'

Reflections

Breaking and accepting bad news may raise many different emotions in individuals and may change family dynamics. Carers often worry as the patient deteriorates over time, and those diagnosed with a terminal illness may find communication is difficult and emotionally draining. It can be incredibly challenging for the patient to manage their own grief alongside that of family members and friends, generating conflicting expectations and a level of guilt. Therefore, a conscious effort was made to sensitively address the emotional state and needs of both Will and his wife. My combined responsibilities of assessing and addressing the emotional and psychological needs of the patient, at the same time as supporting his wife and family, can be stressful, and the complexities of family dynamics may require advanced communication skills.

Noticing emotional cues, facial expressions, and body language is essential in initiating conversations and resolving emotional conflict amicably for both the patient and the spouse. Being truthful and kind are core values that can help alleviate emotional distress and support openness and trust in these conversations. This can be made more difficult when participants are experiencing raw emotions, including a sense of helplessness at being unable to change the situation.

Anger is a common emotion amongst those struggling to cope with terminal illness, often coupled with feelings of guilt and hopelessness. It is crucial to help distressed carers express their anger, frustration, or feelings of guilt and betrayal, and find resolution. Using appropriate communication skills and techniques such as using mirroring and paying attention to non-verbal cues may help alleviate psychological distress. Asking open-ended questions whilst supporting truth-telling with gentleness and kindness can help individuals move towards resolving their feelings.

Discussing death evokes negative emotions, including despondency, and may challenge a person's spirituality and beliefs, causing internal conflict. It is important that whilst acknowledging the situation, we understand that we cannot improve the situation. My role here is to provide support rather than to make the patient better because Will's circumstances cannot be changed. Instead, I seek to ensure that the patient and his family feel valued, respected, and heard.

Denial is a common response to the bad news which health professionals sometimes need to communicate to patients and their families. Blocking behaviours and avoidance behaviours which may be observed include occasions when the person seeks to normalise or minimise the situation with stereotyped comments, such as 'I'm sure it will be fine.' Healthcare professionals need to be wary of giving inappropriate advice, asking leading questions, using closed questions, or asking multiple questions at once, all of which can be ways of avoiding talking about strong feelings. Other blocking strategies that could be either deliberately or inadvertently used due to feeling emotional discomfort are the use of delaying tactics or shifting responsibility for telling the truth to someone else, such as suggesting that more difficult questions are kept for the doctor at a later point. Engaging in superficial chit-chat, jollying along with the patient and their carer or changing the subject, whilst selectively attending to specific cues which feel emotionally safer, or even becoming defensive, are all ways of avoiding difficult conversations.

In summary, this case study demonstrates how important it is for health professionals to use their softer skills, such as verbal and non-verbal communication skills, to deliver person-centred care and facilitate difficult conversations with patients and their families.

Questions for reflection and discussion

Explore the key issues raised in the above scenario as you answer the following six questions:

1. Psychological problems are common among patients living with cancer. Why is it also important to recognise their prevalence amongst carers and family members?

2. There are six widely recognised non-verbal communication skills: facial expressions, eye contact, posture, gestures, touch, and personal space. Identify which of these non-verbal communication skills the nurse uses in her interaction with Mary and Will? Were they appropriate to the situation or not?

3. What are the key attitudes and behaviours a health practitioner may find helpful in delivering bad news? How can these help a person transition to understand that an illness is life-threatening?

4. Patients often drop hints or cues about underlying issues. Identify the kinds of communication skills needed to effectively notice and respond to these cues.

5. Empathy is used to encourage patients or carers to explore their feelings more deeply. In what ways is empathy an appropriate skill to use when delivering bad news?

6. Reflect on the impact of health practitioners using blocking behaviours to protect either themselves or the person in front of them from distress.

Further reading

Curtis, J.R., Back, A.L., Ford, D.W., Downey, L., Shannon, S.E., Doorenbos, A.Z., Kross, E.K., Reinke, L.F., Feemster, L.C., Edlund, B. and Arnold, R.W. (2013) Effect of communication skills training for residents and nurse practitioners on quality of communication with patients with serious illness: A randomized trial. *JAMA*, 310(21): 62271–62281.

Ekman, P. (1992) An argument for basic emotions. *Cognition & Emotion*, 6(3–4): 169–200.

Farsides, C., Higginson, I., Monroe, B., Wilkinson, S., Leliopoulou, C., Costantini, M., Toscani, F., Batiste, X. and Zylicz, B. (2001) Conducting theory with an eye to practice. *European Journal of Palliative Care*, 3.

Orford, N.R., Milnes, S., Simpson, N., Keely, G., Elderkin, T., Bone, A., Martin, P., Bellomo, R., Bailey, M. and Corke, C. (2019) Effect of communication skills training on outcomes in critically ill patients with life-limiting illness referred for intensive care management: A before-and-after study. *BMJ Supportive & Palliative Care*, 9(1): e21–e21.

Stroebe, M., Schut, H. and Stroebe, W. (2005) Attachment in coping with bereavement: A theoretical integration. *Review of General Psychology*, 9(1): 48–66.

Further information

VALUES

Truth-telling involves sharing facts openly without causing unnecessary harm or diminishing hope and is fundamental to the communication skills of palliative care teams. As well as telling the truth when delivering bad news, it is also important to incorporate cultural competence to ensure that the information is conveyed in a way which respects the patient's cultural background and beliefs.

THEORIES

Closed awareness means that the person who is dying does not know or suspect that fact, but the family is aware and chooses not to disclose. There are several awareness contexts or social interactions, according to Glaser and Strauss (2017), between those who are dying and those around the dying. Other contexts are 'suspected awareness,' 'mutual pretence,' and 'open awareness.'

Coping strategies explain how different individuals may perceive situations differently and how coping approaches may impact on the individual's well-being or their ability to manage stress and anxiety. Individual characteristics often play a significant role in the way they react or express emotions such as fear and anger. Lazarus and Folkman's Transactional Model of Stress and Coping (1987) helps us understand how individuals evaluate sources of stress and respond to them in their environment. Similarly, the Dual Process Model of Coping (Larsen et al., 2025) provides insight into how people manage grief whilst continuing with everyday life, suggesting that oscillation between actively grieving and engaging in distraction or avoidance can help with successful adjustment.

Despondency refers to situations in which psychological and spiritual concerns around feelings and thoughts of hopelessness, death anxiety, and loss of dignity have become overwhelming. Interventions designed to improve communication, understanding, and reconciliation within the family during conflicts may alleviate feelings of despondency.

Disease progression in palliative care involves assessing and treating psychological distress, as well as managing physical symptoms such as pain, using both pharmacological and non-pharmacological methods.

End-of-life care includes providing information of what to expect in the final phase of their disease so that both patients and their families can plan care for during this stage, if they choose to do so. Death and dying theories are helpful to enable us to understand the biological, psychological, and spiritual needs of the dying person and their loved ones as they approach the end-of-life.

Hopelessness is a feeling or state of despair. Hopelessness, by definition, is the belief that things are not going to get better or that you cannot succeed in bringing about change for the better.

Suspected awareness arises when the person who is ill begins to suspect that more is going on than is being said (Glaser and Strauss, 2017).

APPROACHES

Empathy is the ability to imagine what someone else may be feeling. It can encourage patients and carers to explore their feelings more deeply, helping them gain a clearer insight into their experiences and emotions. Empathy, alongside warmth and genuineness, provides the basis for a supportive relationship known as the 'therapeutic triad' (Guerin, 1996).

Managing strong emotions is about enabling individuals to reconnect with how they feel, improving communication with self and others, enhancing feelings of control and accepting strong feelings.

Mirroring is a psychological technique often used in counselling, which is used to build rapport with another person.

Misdiagnosis and mistreatment refer to issues in medical and nursing practice, which may delay appropriate treatment. These errors carry significant moral, ethical, and psychological consequences for patients and their families, as well as for professionals.

MODELS

Breaking bad news is usually done using models to help healthcare professionals facilitate difficult conversations. For example, the SPIKES model (Baile et al., 2000) stands for setting up, perception, invitation, knowledge; emotions with empathy, strategy, and summary, offering a structured approach to communicate news to patients.

Communication skills both verbal and non-verbal are foundational to healthcare provision. These skills are used to convey values such as integrity, respect, compassion, courtesy, and sensitivity to the comfort and dignity needs of patients and their families (Gambles et al., 2001; Wilkinson et al., 2001; Wilkinson et al., 2003). Universal facial expressions refer to the non-verbal expression of the seven basic human emotions recognisable across cultures (contempt, happiness, anger, disgust, surprise, fear and sadness – known as CHADsurFs). The term was coined by psychologist Paul Ekman (1992). Soler Model is a non-verbal communication model and refers to the context set up for communicating news to the patient. SOLER stands for sitting squarely, open posture, leaning towards the other, eye contact, and relaxation. The model argues that these conditions ensure a calm and relaxed environment for the patient and health practitioner to exchange information and opinions about diagnoses and treatments (Egan, 1990).

Stages of grief are a model put forward by Kübler-Ross and Kessler (2014) explaining the various stages a person may go through before they accept a situation or outcome (denial, anger, bargaining, depression, and acceptance).

References

Baile, W.F., Buckman, R., Lenzi, R., Glober, G., Beale, E.A. and Kudelka, A.P. (2000) SPIKES – A six-step protocol for delivering bad news: Application to the patient with cancer. *Oncologist*, 5(4): 302–311. doi: 10.1634/theoncologist.5-4-302. PMID: 10964998.

Egan, G. (1990) *The skilled helper: A systematic approach to effective helping*. Thomson Brooks/Cole Publishing Co.

Ekman, P. (1992) Facial expressions of emotion: An old controversy and new findings. *Philosophical Transactions of the Royal Society of London. Series B: Biological Sciences*, 335(1273): 63–69.

Gambles, M., Leliopoulou, C., Roberts, A. and Wilkinson, S. (2001) The long and short of communication skills training: A qualitative evaluation and comparison of participant perceptions of two approaches to communication skill training. *European Journal of Cancer*, 37(Supp 6): S410.

Glaser, B.G. and Strauss, A.L. (2017) *Awareness of dying*. Routledge.

Guerin, P.J. (1996) *Working with relationship triangles: The one-two-three of psychotherapy.* Guilford Press.

Kübler-Ross, E. and Kessler, D. (2014) *On grief and grieving: Finding the meaning of grief through the five stages of loss.* Simon and Schuster.

Larsen, L.H., Hybholt, L. and O'Connor, M. (2025) Lived experience and the dual process model of coping with bereavement: A participatory research study. *Death Studies*, 49(6): 743–754.

Lazarus, R.S. and Folkman, S. (1987) Transactional theory and research on emotions and coping. *European Journal of Personality*, 1(3): 141–169.

Wilkinson, S., Fellowes, D. and Leliopoulou, C. (2001) Does telling the truth about diagnosis and prognosis affect patients' psychological distress? A systematic review registered with the York Centre for Research & Dissemination database. In *The 2001 British Psychosocial Oncology Society Annual Conference*, 11(6): 558. 81wv2.

Wilkinson, S.M., Leliopoulou, C., Gambles, M. and Roberts, A. (2003) Can intensive three-day programmes improve nurses' communication skills in cancer care? *Psycho-Oncology: Journal of the Psychological, Social and Behavioral Dimensions of Cancer*, 12(8): 747–759.

Case study 15
Ben: when options run out

Helen Humphrey and Marie O'Donovan

Referral to paediatric palliative care service

I meet Ben and his parents whilst working as a paediatric palliative care nurse specialist. A referral has been made for symptom management and parallel planning by the oncology nurse specialist at the regional tertiary centre. Ben is 5 years old and has a progression of a brain tumour known as a diffuse intrinsic pontine glioma (DIPG). Ben's parents have consented to a referral to the paediatric palliative care service, and we are invited to join a clinic appointment with Ben's oncologist. The purpose of this appointment is for a clinical review after completing radiotherapy and to introduce the process of parallel planning, symptom management, and hospice services.

APPROACH: parallel planning

MODEL: palliative care

Clinic appointment

Athena, the Oncology Nurse Specialist, invites me into the clinic appointment where Ben's parents (Vince and Linda) and his lead oncologist are present. I am told Ben has remained on the ward with his grandparents. Athena introduces me, saying, 'Vince and Linda, this is Kira, who is a clinical nurse specialist within the hospice team.' From the family's body language and facial expressions, I realise that they are uncomfortable with my introduction. Mum has her arms folded and does not appear to want to make eye contact with me. Dad does make some eye contact with me, his face appearing serious and somewhat stern. I follow on from my introduction saying, 'Thank you Athena, good to meet you both. I'm joining the appointment today, following on from the referral Dr Malik discussed with you, to find out about how Ben and you are as a family, and to talk with you about services that are available to you as a family. Is that okay with you both?' I sit directly opposite

APPROACH: multi-professional teamworking

DOI: 10.4324/9781003651758-15

Linda and Vince, at their level, and speak clearly whilst maintaining eye contact.

Linda looks flushed, and for a few moments, the room remains silent. After a whilst, she speaks: 'I have to be honest with you, I don't believe my son is going to die. I'm part of a DIPG family forum and have found a treatment which we have begun fundraising for.' Vince then seeks to clarify this as he adds, 'But we do understand that you are here to help with Ben's symptoms, like his headaches and vomiting.'

At first, I am taken a back by the force of Linda's statement but reflect that she is probably feeling scared, so I endeavour to make the conversation feel safer, saying,

'Thank you for being honest with us; we understand how difficult it is to have these conversations. Can I ask more about the treatment you are referring to, please? Can you

tell me what you understand it to involve and where it would take place?'

Linda calms a little and gets out her notebook whilst saying, 'It's intraventricular chemotherapy, which we believe will be a cure for Ben's cancer. This would be abroad. Have you heard of it?' She shows me information about a trial I have some knowledge of. I therefore share further information with them: 'I am aware that there are some international phase 1 trials currently underway for this treatment. There were some treatment centres within the UK in the past,

but these have closed, and I'm unsure of the reason why. Do you understand what a phase 1 trial is and what this treatment would involve?'

Vince answers, 'Yes, we do, and we have been provided with information from the trial team, after a virtual consult-ation with them.'

I am reassured that they do have some knowledge and information, but feel it is worth exploring in more depth, so ask, 'I want to ensure that you understand that the purpose of a phase 1 trial is not a curative treatment, but a means of exploring the impact of the drug on the patient's body - its

safety and side effects.'

Parents in need

Linda appears visibly distressed and tearful as she replies, 'We will do anything to save Ben, and we don't believe he is going to die.' Vince adds, 'We love our son, and we have to know that we have done everything we can to make him well.'

It is clear to me that this is a family in distress and experiencing grief, so recognising that it is important to acknowledge this, I respond, 'I really do appreciate how difficult this is and thank you for being open and honest with us. It's important that we work together to manage Ben's cancer and knowing what information you are exploring elsewhere is important to ensure the safety of decisions that we make, such as in managing Ben's symptoms. I'd like to explore Ben's current symptoms and how he is right now, is that okay? Once we've reviewed Ben together, it would be good to discuss with you the potential risks of Ben travelling abroad, especially if this involves flying.'

VALUE: transparency

APPROACH: professional advocacy

Linda continues to be tearful. Vince answers, 'Yes, that's fine, we think he has been doing well after finishing radiotherapy and completing steroids.'

I can see from Linda's facial expression that she is finding the conversation was difficult, but due to Vince's engaging manner, I continue to explore the situation with them. 'I'd also like to meet Ben, if that's okay with you both Can you tell me what you are aware of Ben's understanding of his diagnosis?'

THEORY: consent

APPROACH: professional curiosity

Vince again answers, 'We've told him that his brain is poorly, and that he needs to spend some time in the hospital for the doctors and nurses to make him better, but he will get better.'

Mum then adds, 'We don't want him to know or to worry about what is happening.'

Having this information, I consider it important to ask: 'Do you think it's likely that Ben will ask me questions about what is happening?'

APPROACH: professional curiosity

Linda replies, 'I don't think he'll ask you anything, he is usually very quiet with strangers.'

I am not surprised by this, so continue, 'That's understandable, can I discuss with you what we might say if Ben asks questions beyond what you've already told him. There is lots of guidance available to support you both to have an open conversations with Ben or to respond to questions he may have.'

Ben's symptoms

I enquire further: 'I understand at Ben's diagnosis he presented with morning vomiting, severe headaches and poor coordination, which may have been referred to as ataxia at the time. Is that right?'

Dad responds by saying, 'Yes that's right, he also had a facial palsy, particularly of his right eyelid - I can't remember what they called this, it had a special word.' I realise I know what he is referring to, so I say, 'Ah, the word may have been ptosis? Vince nods, affirming that this was the word used. I go on to say, 'Can you tell me about Ben's vomiting and headaches since completing radiotherapy?'

Vince looks at Linda, who replies, 'It's not been so bad; he does occasionally still vomit and have headaches.'

APPROACH: professional curiosity

I continue: 'Can you tell me how frequently Ben is vomiting and when this happens?'.

Mum refers to her notebook, saying, 'Most mornings, but it's only a little bit and he feels better afterwards.'

I go on to ask, 'When will this be? Is there a normal time, such as on waking, moving, or sitting up?' To which mum responds, 'Usually on waking, when he first gets up.'

I can see that Linda's posture has relaxed, and she is now engaging with me and giving eye contact. I think this is probably because we are focusing on Ben's symptoms and not the prognosis or treatment, so I continue. 'Okay, thank you, it's good to be clear on the frequency and when this is happening. You say it's only a small amount, can you tell be approximately how much – such as a small cup full (approx. 150 mls) or a 50 p size vomit, as well as the colour and consistency?'

Mum replies, 'It's yellowy white and looks like phlegm but it's probably about half a small cup full. He always feels better afterwards.'

I continue to engage in this line of conversation, 'That's really helpful to know. Does Ben tell you that he feels sick at any other times during the day?'

Mum again refers to her notebook and then confirms, 'He felt sick at the beginning of radiotherapy, but this settled with the steroids and doesn't seem to have come back.'

I am reassured through this conversation with Linda that she will be open to working with me and that we will be able to develop a therapeutic relationship. As I am listening to and acknowledging her extensive knowledge of Ben's symptoms, I continue with, 'I'm glad to hear that the steroids helped manage his nausea and this currently doesn't appear to be a problem. We anticipate that the symptoms Ben experienced at diagnosis and during treatment, like vomiting and headaches, may return as Ben's disease progresses and he is no longer on steroids, so it's important that we monitor this. Did you notice any other symptoms whilst Ben was on steroids such as changes in mood, behaviour, or appetite?'

THEORY: parent-nurse partnership

APPROACH: education

APPROACH: symptom management

Vince then shares, 'He would be quite tearful especially around bedtime but couldn't tell me why.'

I acknowledge, 'That must be really difficult to see and upsetting for you both.'

Linda cuts in, saying, 'It is but, as we've said, it all seems to have settled since stopping the steroids.'

It is apparent from her tone that Linda does not want to discuss Ben's emotional state, so I decide to continue to focus the conversation on his symptom management: 'Can you tell me about his headaches: how frequent they are and what happens?'

Linda's tone of voice settles, and her body appears to relax as she says, 'Initially before radiotherapy he had them every day, multiple times during the day, intense pain and they would wake him during the night. I think they're now roughly every other day, about once a day, he'll scream and hold his head and will lay himself down, which seems to help.'

I realise this is a significant symptom, and we will need to explore this further. 'Thank you, Linda, that's really important to know, could you give me an idea how long it usually takes Ben to recover from these episodes, and whether you give him anything for them?'

Linda replies, 'It depends, sometimes he'll lay on the sofa for about an hour. I was giving him a dose of Oramorph and Paracetamol which seemed to help but they seem to be clearing quicker now.'

Vince interjects, 'The one the other day lasted about 4 hours; he was really grumpy afterwards.'

'But that was the first one for weeks that's lasted more than an hour,' Linda impatiently responds.

I note the atmosphere between Linda and Vince shift and feel it would be useful to step in here. 'I can see that this is varied. I can see you are already using a notebook, so it would be really useful if you could continue to keep a record of Ben's symptoms such as his headaches - when they happen, what Ben does, how long it lasts, whether anything seems to trigger the headache, whether you give him any medication, what you give and did it help? It's useful for us to look at patterns of symptoms, potential triggers, what works and what doesn't to manage them, so we can consider how we might manage symptoms with such things as buccal medication for flash headache. Buccal is like an oral medication which is placed between the child's gum and cheek and is absorbed there, instead of him needing to swallow it. This way in bypasses the stomach and can often take affect quicker than oral morphine.'

Mum seems interested in this, and her posture becomes more open as she leans forward, making eye contact with me as she says, 'That would be useful, as he is sometimes sick when taking his medication, and he hates them really.' However, Linda's demeanour changes again as she pulls back and folds her arms, saying, 'But I do worry that we seem to be focusing on his disease getting worse, which we don't want to do. It feels like we're giving up on him.'

Sensitive discussions

I can see that this is a difficult thought for mum, so I say, 'We know that it's upsetting to talk about symptoms and disease progression. Let me reassure you that we are not giving up on Ben. Our aim is to work together to support you and manage Ben's symptoms appropriately.'

Both Linda and Vince remain silent and don't answer for a few moments. The room is quiet. Vince eventually states with an abrupt tone, 'It feels as though all the things we want to do to give Ben the best chance of getting well, you say we can't do, or it won't work. We don't believe our son is going to die, didn't you hear us the first time?'

We are reaching the end of Linda and Vince's tolerance level for discussing this with me, so I gently say, 'I apologise if I've upset either of you; that's not been our intention. As I said our aim is always to work together to support you as a family and to ensure that Ben remains well and stable for as long as possible, but also to be open and honest with you both'. They both remain still, Linda looks down at the floor and Vince looks at me, so I speak mostly to him as I add, 'Shall we have a break as I'm conscious we've discussed a lot already. Before we finish our meeting today, the consultant and I would like to explain to you our concerns around the potential risks of Ben travelling, especially by air. I'd also like to say hello to Ben if that's okay with you.'

Mum looks up at me with a start and says, 'We don't want you to see him on your own, we'll be with him too and we'll need to decide who we tell him you are and where you're from.'

I can see Linda's distress in her wide eyes so reassure her by saying, 'That really is all okay, you can tell him I'm a nurse who works with Athena and Dr Malik and has just come to say hello to you.' Mum gives a little nod at this again, her posture appeared to relax into the chair again, so I continue, 'I really do understand your apprehension about using the word hospice and the ideas this brings to mind for lots of people. Most families I've worked with are initially apprehensive, but the hospice is about much more than death and dying. It's about working with and supporting you as a family and as individuals, accessing services such as play and music therapy, counselling, opportunities to make memories and have new experiences supported by hospice staff and to have access to the specialist nurse team 24 hours a day, seven days a week. You are welcome to visit and have lunch at the hospice and have a look round as a family, if you'd like to at any point.'

APPROACH: compassionate communication

Vince looks at Linda, who appears to be looking at the floor again, and says, 'We'll consider it in the future but for now it's not our focus.'

I reply warmly, 'I understand that, thank you for allowing me to tell you more about the services available to you. Before we finish today, I'll leave you with our contact details, in case you would like to come and have a look around.'

Reflections

The diagnosis of DIPG was devastating for Ben's parents, who are struggling to process the gravity of the situation. DIPG is known for its poor prognosis, with most patients surviving less than a year from the time of diagnosis. The reality that there are no standard curative treatments available is overwhelming for Ben's parents, who are not yet ready to accept the terminal nature of their child's illness.

Denial and hope for a cure have driven them to seek a second opinion and to consider participation in experimental research trials. Additionally, they have started raising funds for unsupported medical treatment abroad, demonstrating their desperation and hope of finding a solution, however slim the chances may be. The presence of social media, crowdfunding, and public fundraising campaigns have become commonplace, but also bring their own ethical dilemmas.

End-of-life and parallel planning conversations are, of course, something that no parent or family wants to have, but openness around symptomology and end-of-life care is, on occasion, welcomed by families.

As the nurse specialist working with Ben's family, this situation presents several ethical challenges for the healthcare team, particularly for the nurse specialist who is providing ongoing support to the family. The family's inability to accept the prognosis and their pursuit of alternative treatments create tension and stress within the multidisciplinary team. The lead consultant and I must balance empathy for the family's emotional turmoil with the need to provide realistic information about the likely outcomes and the limitations of available treatments, as well as continuing a professional relationship with the family.

The niche speciality of children and young people's oncology within geographical areas and specialist treatment centres brings together many families who may have some similar and some different experiences in treatments, responses to treatments, and side effects. Naturally, families will often gravitate towards one another, join forums or use social media to share experiences and to access support (Nagelhout et al., 2018). This can both support and divide; therefore, demanding professionalism from the multidisciplinary team.

The family's plan to seek medical treatment abroad and their efforts to raise funds add another layer of complexity. The specialist nurse is faced with the ethical dilemma of supporting the family's wishes whilst knowing that these unsupported treatments may offer false hope and could potentially cause more harm than good. The pressure on the multidisciplinary team to approve Ben as fit to travel, despite his clinical instability, is also a significant concern. Flying in his current condition could exacerbate his symptoms or lead to life-threatening complications, highlighting a potential conflict between the family's wishes and Ben's best interests.

The level of uncertainty within paediatric palliative care is often one of the biggest challenges; however, the role of compassionate communication is fundamental in developing therapeutic relationships with children, young people, and their families, despite the uncertainty (Gault et al., 2017). The importance of allowing families time to talk and listen, and for them to feel heard is imperative even when their decision-making and thought processes differ from the team's recommendations. The importance of active listening, engagement, and awareness of the importance of both verbal and non-verbal communication is at the very centre of providing quality holistic nursing care.

The nurse's role is multifaceted, requiring a combination of clinical expertise, emotional intelligence, and ethical sensitivity. By providing compassionate support and accurate information and advocating for Ben's best interests, the nurse can help guide the family through this difficult journey, ensuring that Ben's remaining time is as comfortable and as meaningful as possible.

Questions for reflection and discussion

Explore the key issues raised in the above scenario as you answer the following six questions:

1. How can health professionals best manage prognostic uncertainty when talking to children, young people, adults, and their families with life-limiting and life-threatening conditions?

2. In what ways can principles of palliative care, such as parallel planning and symptom management, be normalised as part of standard care?

3. What are the best approaches to introducing parents and families to palliative care services and to discussing referral?

4. Consider the challenges of discussing professional concerns with parents and families, such as accessing experimental treatment, use of unlicensed medications, and air or foreign travel.

5. Consider how we can ensure channels of communication remain open between health practitioners and families in cases where disagreement has impacted the professional relationship.

6. How important is it to consider the understanding and knowledge that children and young people have about their diagnosis? To what extent is it a necessary concern for professionals?

Further reading

Barrett. L., Fraser, L., Noyes, J., Taylor, J. and Hackett, J. (2023) Understanding Parent Experiences of End-of-Life Care for Children: A Systematic Review and Qualitative Evidence Synthesis. *Palliative Medicine*, 37(2): 178–202. Available at: doi: 10.1177/02692163221144084.

Children and Young People's Advance Care Plan (2023) *Collaborative Planning for End-of-Life Decisions. Best Practice Guidelines to Enhance the Process of Advanced Care Planning for a Child or Young Person.* Available at: https://cypacp.uk/wp-content/uploads/2023/11/CYPACP-Guidance-Nov-2023.pdf. (Accessed 30th September 2024).

European Association for Palliative Care (2022) *European Charter on Palliative Care for Children and Young People* Available at: https://eapcnet.eu/eapc-groups/reference/children-young-people/ (Accessed 5th October 2024).

Fraser, L.K., Gibson-Smith, D., Jarvis, S., Norman, P. and Parslow, R. (2020) Make Every Child Count Estimating Current and Future Prevalence of Children and Young People with Life-Limiting Conditions in the United Kingdom. *Palliative Medicine*, 35(9): 1641–1651. Available at: doi: 10.1177/0269216320975308.

Scott, H.M., Coombes, L., Braybrook, D., Harðardóttir, D., Roach, A., Brislowe, L., Bluebond-Langmer, M, Fraser, L., Downing, J., Farsides, B., Murtagh, F.E.M., Ellis-Smith, C. and Harding, R. (2024) What Are the Anticipated Benefits, Risks, Barriers and Facilitators to Implementing Person-Centred Outcome Measures into Routine Care for Children and Young People with Life-Limiting and Life-Threatening Conditions? A Qualitative Interview Study with Key Stakeholders. *Palliative Medicine*, 38(4): 471–484. doi: 10.1177/02692163241234797.

Further information

VALUES

Honesty is an essential quality in any person working in healthcare due to the vulnerability of service users, many of whom will be living with long-term conditions, which may make them fully or partially dependent on the care and support of others.

Transparency is openness and accountability, not just when things go wrong but when the outcome is unknown, to ensure safe and effective nursing care. It includes learning from errors and an openness to share this not only with colleagues but with service users.

THEORIES

Consent recognises the importance of informed and valid consent to treatment and procedures and involves providing information and explaining issues such as process, side effects, benefits, and risks in a form that is accessible and comprehensible.

Parent-nursing partnerships recognise that parents or main caregivers can have deep insights into their child's normal behaviours, comfort levels, and needs and can identify subtle changes in symptoms that nurses or other healthcare professionals may not immediately notice. Their involvement ensures that care is aligned with the child's preferences and personality. Parents should be seen as key partners in care planning and making treatment-based decisions. Nurses provide nursing expertise, whilst parents bring intimate knowledge of their children. Together, they create a strong, supportive care team.

Stigma relating to the experiences and impact of cancer on children, young people and their families is often wide-ranging and can include the wider family, friends, acquaintances, schools, and communities. There remain misconceptions around diagnosis, treatment, and survival.

APPROACHES

Active listening is central to building therapeutic relationships by allowing children, young people, adults, and their families time and opportunities to speak and be heard.

Compassionate communication is an approach that includes active listening, recognising the importance of both non-verbal and verbal communication, and being empathetic.

Confidence is an important element of communication in decision-making, with clarity being able to share and explain and provide rationale but also being able to explain risk or uncertainty.

Education about symptoms and disease progression helps parents prepare emotionally and practically for what to expect. This helps them make informed choices about interventions, hospice care, and end-of-life preferences. It ensures the child has a peaceful, dignified, and comfortable experience, surrounded by love.

Empathy is essential for providing person-centred care. It enables the person providing support to better understand the world from the perspective of the patient and, therefore, to respond to their experience of service delivery with an individualised approach.

Information gathering is a key aspect of decision-making, gathering, and reviewing information to inform and support decisions.

Multi-professional teamworking is an essential aspect of providing high-quality care, as each professional brings unique expertise, skills, and tools to the team.

Non-verbal communication includes gestures, facial expressions, movements, eye contact, and posture, alongside the volume, tone, and pitch of speech and vocalisations. Each person has an individual profile of non-verbal communication, although there may be some culturally and socially derived gestures and expressions which people from similar backgrounds share.

Parallel planning is an essential part of the organisation and delivery of palliative care. It is the planning for the unexpected, the what ifs, to ensure safe and effective care.

Professional advocacy is ensuring that patient outcomes are safeguarded, championing the rights of the child, young person, adult, and family to promote high-quality, safe, and effective care.

Professional curiosity is at the heart of safe and effective nursing care, being continually curious by asking, listening, questioning, and reflecting to protect patient outcomes.

Symptom management is the focus of care around presenting symptoms and considering pharmacological and non-pharmacological management.

MODELS

Child/family-centred care is the approach of holding the child, young person, and their family at the centre of everything we do, involving them in decision-making, planning, and care delivery, whilst continually exploring their hopes, wishes, and preferences.

Palliative care is a total and holistic approach to care for children, young people, adults, and their families with life-limiting and life-threatening conditions. It should focus as much on living, hopes, wishes, preferences, and priorities as it does on death, dying, and bereavement.

References

Gault, I., Shapcott, J., Luthi, A. and Reid, G. (2017) *Communication in Nursing and Healthcare: A Guide for Compassionate Practice.* Sage: London.

Nagelhout, E.S., Linder, L.A., Austin, T., Parsons, B.G., Scott, B., Gardner, E., Spraker-Perlman, H., Verma, A., Fluchel, M.N. and Wu, Y.P. (2018) Social Media Use among Parents and Caregivers of Children with Cancer. *Journal of Pediatric Oncology Nursing.* 35(6): 399–405. doi: 10.1177/1043454218795091.

Case study 16
Gareth: until we meet again?

Sarah Housden

The chaplain is called

The role of a hospital chaplain provides opportunities to come alongside people of many different faiths, as well as those without any formal or even informal expression of faith. It is not necessarily of primary importance to me what people believe in terms of their religious traditions, as I want to be able to walk with individuals as they seek meaning in the unique experiences, past and present, which life has brought to them. Supporting patients and their families through some of the loneliest and most desolate times of their lives, as well as through experiences of joy and peace, all mixed in with feelings of hope and fear, draws upon my firmly held belief in the worth of every human life, more than on my personal faith in a particular formalised expression of faith or in a specific understanding of the nature of God. Whilst this may not be the case for every hospital chaplain, it is this approach that, for me, enables me to work with people of diverse spiritual and non-spiritual backgrounds.

MODEL: chaplaincy

MODEL: multi-faith chaplaincy

VALUE: compassion

VALUE: valuing people

VALUE: caring

APPROACH: non-judgemental

VALUE: acceptance

One of my foremost observations in this work is the spiritual or existential pain, which can occur in serious illness if patients are unable to find meaning in their experience. Similarly, situations of significant challenge in my work occurs where emotional and spiritual discord are experienced due to the incongruence between strongly held beliefs in a good and all-powerful God who can intervene and bring healing in the presence of no such healing.

THEORY: total pain

VALUE: understanding

Gareth is a patient whom I have been asked to speak with by ward staff because of what seems to be his denial of his worsening ill health despite having a prognosis of a very limited remaining lifespan. The first thing I need to clarify is whether Gareth himself wants to see a chaplain.

APPROACH: consent

DOI: 10.4324/9781003651758-16

Meeting Gareth

Gareth is 70 years old and is one of the leaders of a well-known independent faith-based group, which meets in our local town and has a well-established history of supporting the homeless, those in poverty and many others in difficult life situations. The group is well-respected locally amongst people from a wide range of religious traditions, and I am familiar with Gareth from ecumenical and interfaith meetings which I have attended over the past 15 years.

As I approach Gareth's area of the ward, I see that he has a visitor, so I plan to introduce myself quickly and arrange to return later if that is something he would like. Gareth is seated in bed, with several carefully arranged pillows supporting him to sit upright. He looks physically weak, but his smile is radiant as he sees me approaching.

THEORY: non-verbal communication

'Hello, Gareth. My name is Penny and I'm from the chaplaincy team. I am just on the ward visiting a few people this afternoon, and one of the nursing staff mentioned that you might be someone who would like a chat. I can see you are busy right now, but I just wanted to introduce myself and let you know that I or anyone from the team would be very happy to talk with you if that would be something you might like.'

VALUE: communication

Gareth replies slowly, sounding as though he is struggling for breath: *'That's very kind Penny. Thank you. I do have plenty of people visiting who bring me good cheer from a faith perspective, so please don't feel the need to worry about me.'* Gareth goes on to tell me that he does not believe his current illness will end in death and that he has a strong spiritual assurance that he will be healed. I listen attentively, noting his confidence with some degree of admiration. At the same time, I cannot help noticing the body language of his visitor, whose discomfort appears to suggest that she does not share his confidence in his forthcoming recovery.

APPROACH: prayer for healing

APPROACH: active listening

'I'm sorry to have interrupted your visit, Gareth. Please feel free to ask for me at any time should your needs change and do let your family and friends know that they can drop

into the faith centre should they want to talk or pray with anyone.' I share this information with Gareth for the benefit of his visitor, explaining how the hospital faith centre can be reached, whilst expecting that it is unlikely to be Gareth who ultimately needs these directions.

A family in need

Having worked in hospital chaplaincy for several years, there have been many occasions when I have been able to provide a listening ear for patients' family members and friends, sometimes alongside the patient and sometimes separately. There are times when people unexpectedly and unpredictably come to see me at the faith centre after a brief introduction in a clinical environment, and it is no surprise to me when Gareth's visitor comes looking for me shortly after I leave the ward. I welcome her and offer her a seat. She seems more anxious than she had in Gareth's presence, and I wait a moment for her to settle. I want to avoid making assumptions about why she has come and what she wants to say.

THEORY: avoiding assumptions

'My Dad must not know that I've come to see you, Penny. Please promise me you won't tell him.' Mindful of the strict guidance around as well as limits on confidentiality, I swiftly assure her that our conversation will remain confidential between us unless I have a cause for concern which needs reporting elsewhere. Her nod tells me that she understands and is probably familiar with the boundaries of confidential conversations in both faith- and hospital-based settings.

APPROACH: confidentiality

'I'm Ruth. My Dad – Gareth – you see he is a man of immense faith, and in his time, he has seen some wonderful answers to prayer, including all kinds of healings from physical and psychological conditions as well as people being set free from terrible life circumstances. There are so many stories that he can tell you. But ....' She pauses and I wait for her to go on, nodding slightly to give her some non-verbal encouragement.

APPROACH: prayer

'The thing is, Penny, that my Mum died twenty-five years ago and he wouldn't accept that she was going to die, so

APPROACH: realism

none of us were prepared for it when she did die. We were all still praying for her healing as she lay dead in the next room, because he didn't tell us she had gone, because he would not accept it. I was just twenty-three. Losing a parent, or anyone, to cancer is so awful, but never having had the chance to say goodbye is heartbreaking. Goodness knows what Mum went through when she saw the end approaching and couldn't say her goodbyes to us, her children, because of Dad's complete assurance of her imminent healing. I'm not saying either way whether healings can happen – that's not something I want to discuss. I just cannot stand to lose another parent without being able to let them go gently. I need to prepare for what is happening and he is not letting me do that'.

THEORY: loss

THEORY: perspectives on reality

Despite the urgency in her tone, the residual grief about losing her mother and a strong hint of frustration or even anger towards her father, Ruth maintains her composure throughout what she says. She is not tearful, but at the end of telling me this, she does take a long breath in, followed by what sounds like a sigh of relief. I wonder whether she has said something to me today that she has not been able to say before.

APPROACH: empathy

APPROACH: therapeutic silence

We sit in silence together for what feels like a few minutes. I am unsure of how best to help Ruth and the other family members in this situation, but I recognise this moment of sharing her feelings about the manner of her mother's death and her fear of the same situation occurring with her father as potentially bringing her some resolution and healing for long-held feelings.

THEORY: emotional healing

Hope for the future

I break the silence as Ruth's breathing settles: '*I'm here for you Ruth, as well as for your father. What would you like to happen now?'*.

APPROACH: shared decision-making

VALUE: sensitivity

MODEL: communities of believers

She turned to me, and her desire for a solution that builds rather than compromises faith is clear. '*I just want me and my two sisters, as well as the wider family of the church community, to have the opportunity to prepare for Dad's death. I want us to be able to experience all the feelings associated with the pain and fear of loss, as well as the hope that we will one day see each other again in a better place where there will be complete healing for us and for the world – no more of this crying and pain, and certainly no more of having to hide my feelings!'*

VALUE: hope

Ruth is quiet for a moment, then continues: *'I have never spoken with my sisters about what happened with Mum, but they both lost a bit of their faith, and one left the church soon afterwards. I just want us to find our way forwards as a family, and as a community of believers, rooted in reality, so that we can go on supporting one another in loving ways through all the ups and downs of life.'*

Ruth's words remind me of something I have recently said to someone else – that being able to trust in the dark times is the richest form of faith.

'Do you think you could speak with any of the other leaders of your church about this Ruth? Or would you like me to?' I ask, recognising the importance of communicating sensitively with them as well as with her sisters to ensure that her father's beliefs are respected, at the same time as their own care and support needs are met.

VALUE: respect

APPROACH: whole person care

Ruth hesitates for a moment but then says, *'There is one of the leaders who used to work in healthcare. I think she would be a good person for me to speak with first. She gave a great talk at one of our meetings recently about the need for good care for the whole of life and to the end of life. She was talking about the value of life and was saying that with good palliative care most people can experience a worthwhile life for the whole of life, and a good death. I think she would understand what I'm saying about wanting to have a proper goodbye with Dad, as well as about his need to accept palliative care.'*

Ruth and I part company with a plan that she will speak to her sisters and to the church leader she has mentioned, coming back to me should she want or need any further support from me as a hospital chaplain. I feel confident that Ruth has taken steps today that will enable her family and the wider community of believers of which she is a part to move to a position where they can receive a different and more extensive kind of healing than the one her father had been hoping for.

Reflections

One way of interpreting the different perspectives in this case study is to consider that Gareth has ignored the harsh reality of a terminal cancer diagnosis, despite the clear evidence of his physical decline. Another way of seeing the situation is that Gareth's well-being depends on his firmly held beliefs and the maintenance of these. Or it might be considered that this is a family like any other, where the pain of an earlier bereavement, having not been spoken of about in the open, has led to a compounding of this historically poor and complex communication in the present situation.

Each person encountering these situations in healthcare contexts will hold their own views about the rights or wrongs of prayer for healing and the role to be played by religious beliefs in bringing hope in the face of death. Whatever interpretive perspective is held, all healthcare staff involved in Gareth's care need to show sensitivity and respect for his religious beliefs and practices, which are likely to have been the focus of much of his family and working life for decades. For healthcare practitioners who do not share a faith perspective, Gareth's belief that he will experience a supernatural healing may seem like some sort of psychological defence mechanism in the context of the difficulty to face reality of worsening health and impending death. However, we know enough about Gareth to be sure that his lifetime of belief is not just some kind of prop for helping him through life's difficulties, as is evident in the way the faith-based group he co-leads is held in respect within the wider local community.

Key skills required by chaplaincy and the wider healthcare team in situations where a patient or their family hold beliefs which are not necessarily shared by those around them include using sensitive communication to establish an empathic understanding of the perspectives held by those seeing the world and the meaning of life, differently to us. In this case, Penny's role is to listen and support Ruth to find her way to actions which will help to bring healing of memories around her mother's death, as well as an opportunity to prepare for her father's death. This needs to be done without making critical judgements about, or jeopardising the faith of the patient and his family.

Questions for reflection and discussion

Explore the key issues raised in the above scenario as you answer the following six questions:

1. Why is it important to maintain self-awareness about our own perspective on the meaning and purpose of life when working with patients from diverse cultural and faith backgrounds?

2. What are the challenges you might experience in supporting people with their own faith and beliefs in healthcare settings where these are either (a) similar to or (b) different from your own?

3. What are some of the distinct roles of members of the chaplaincy team in relation to supporting patients who are terminally ill and approaching death in your work setting?

4. What provision is made in your workplace for supporting the staff team to understand the needs, beliefs and practices of people from diverse faith backgrounds, particularly towards the end of life?

5. In what ways might support from a chaplaincy team member who has a similar faith or philosophical perspective be preferable to some patients and their families compared to the input of someone who can listen and seek to empathise without sharing the same beliefs?

6. What part do (or could) chaplaincy teams play in supporting you and your colleagues in working with cumulative experiences of patients living with cancer diagnoses and the subsequent navigation of multiple journeys of loss and survival?

Further reading

Gawande, A. (2015) *Being Mortal: Illness, Medicine and What Matters in the End*. London: Profile Books Ltd.

Idler, E., Jalloh, M.F., Cochrane, J. and Blevins, J. (2023) Religion as a social force in health: Complexities and contradictions. *BMJ*. 382: e076817 doi:10.1136/bmj-2023-076817.

Murphy, K. and Whorton, B. (eds) (2017) *Chaplaincy in Hospice and Palliative Care*. London: Jessica Kingsley Publishers.

Public Health England (2016) *Faith at the End of Life*. PHE publications gateway number: 2015499. Available at: https://assets.publishing.service.gov.uk/media/5a809fe1e5274a2e8ab5136c/Faith_at_end_of_life_-_a_resource.pdf (Accessed 29th December 2024).

Tomkins, A., Duff, J., Fitzgibbon, A., Karam, A., Mills, E.J., Munnings, K., Smith, S., Rao Seshadri, S., Steinberg, A., Vitillo, R. and Yugi, P. (2015) Controversies in faith and health care. *The Lancet*. 386(10005): 1776–1785.

Further information

VALUES

Acceptance is central to person-centred practice. It sits alongside being non-judgemental and understanding the perspective of the person as a central tenet of working with people living with cancer as they present throughout their illness trajectories. It is key to promoting patient well-being.

Caring involves practitioners engaging in interactions and interventions which focus on the needs of the person within their context. Caring also includes making use of an evidence-based approach to providing the right care, in a timely way, at every stage of life.

Communication is '*central to successful caring relationships and to effective team working. Listening is as important as what we say and do*' (Department of Health, 2012, p. 13).

Compassion is defined in Compassion in Practice as '*how care is given through relationships based on empathy, respect and dignity*' (Department of Health, 2012, p. 13).

Hope has been described as an integral part of being human and is seen as having three main dimensions: firstly, an inner power that enables people to transcend their present situation; secondly, the anticipation of an improved state; and lastly, as a personal experience, centred on our chances of achieving what we want (Antunes et al., 2023).

Respect involves recognising and acknowledging the unconditional value of all people in a way which enables them to maintain their dignity and self-respect.

Sensitivity involves being aware of how another person is feeling. This can mean needing to pay attention to non-verbal communication and facial expressions, especially where a person may be experiencing more difficulty in expressing themselves.

Understanding involves having a sympathetic awareness of another person's thoughts, feelings, and experiences and is central to providing person-centred care, as well as to providing approaches which help to avoid stress and distress for patients of all backgrounds and abilities.

Valuing people regardless of our differences in background, belief, culture, and outlook is fundamental to respectful healthcare delivery. Person-centred interactions that value, acknowledge, and validate the individual make a huge contribution to an individual's well-being.

THEORIES

Avoiding assumptions: Stenhouse (2021, p. 27) states that practitioners 'must treat people as individuals, avoid making assumptions about them, recognise diversity and individual choice, and respect and uphold their dignity and human rights.'

Emotional healing in the spiritual sense is sometimes believed to come alongside physical healing, but equally, can occur separately from this as in the healing of past hurts, which may be experienced where a person forgives another person, or where they are able to allow a sense of supernatural compassion and comfort to enter the memory of a past hurt. Someone's forgiveness of a person who has hurt them involves a kind of spiritual letting go does not suggest that what happened was right or acceptable.

Loss of any kind can be accompanied by a grief response and does not necessarily involve the death of a person close to us. Loss and grief can also be experienced because of losing contact with an important person, object, or stage of one's life or other significant change, such as the diagnosis of a life-limiting illness, as occurs in some cancers. The grief experience has been described as involving five stages of processing loss (Kubler-Ross and Kessler, 2014), although this model has been both built upon and contested by other authors.

Perspectives on reality relate to an approach to understanding of everyday reality in which each person is seen as having a unique perspective, thus recognising that objective truth for events has limits and that no one individual can claim to see or recall the situation precisely as it is experienced by others.

Non-verbal communication includes gestures, facial expressions, movements, muscle tension, and posture, alongside the volume, tone, and pitch of vocalisations. Each person has an individual profile of non-verbal communication, although there may be some culturally and socially derived gestures and expressions which people from similar backgrounds share.

Total pain has been described as pain which encompasses all aspects of the self — including the physical, psychological, social, spiritual, and practical struggles of a person in the context of life-limiting illness (DeForest and Douglas, 2024).

APPROACHES

Active listening is an essential aspect of respecting patients. Becoming an effective listener involves actively engaging with people to make sense of what we see in their body language, in combination with what we hear. We need to hear, consider, and process what is said to us in nursing, and this is never a passive process (Ali, 2018).

Confidentiality is key to gaining the trust of service users across health and social care and is embedded in the professional codes of conduct of most practitioners. However, within the confidentiality policies of most organisations, there will also be a clause on the limits of confidentiality, stating that a person's details will be shared within the team as clinically required for providing services, and beyond the team with external authorities where an issue arises around child or adult safeguarding, and to prevent someone coming to harm.

Consent to an intervention within health and care is a fundamental aspect of respecting the human rights, choices, and decision-making of individuals. Practitioners across the multidisciplinary team should always check for consent before any intervention or interaction.

Empathy is essential for providing person-centred care. It enables the person providing support to better understand the world from the perspective of the patient and, therefore, to respond to their experience of service delivery with an individualised approach.

Non-judgemental approaches within health and social care practice are central to helping practitioners avoid making premature judgements or assumptions, which could impact professional decision-making and so affect future actions and care planning in detrimental ways (Nibbelink and Brewer, 2018).

Prayer is seen differently within different traditions, and in some religious traditions, there are several distinct types of prayer. Within many faith traditions, prayer is seen as talking with God and can involve asking him to meet a range of needs, including for healing from past hurts, present psychological or physical needs or other difficult life circumstances. Some faith traditions will use more formalised pre-written and authorised prayers, whilst others will use more spontaneous approaches to communicating with God.

Prayer for healing is undertaken by people from a variety of faith backgrounds and may involve a person praying for their own healing or asking others to pray for them. In the latter scenario, there may be physical contact between the prayer and the prayed-for person, as well as the use of sanctified anointing oils.

Realism is a key part of providing effective and evidence-based healthcare provision for practitioners. It involves a combination of acceptance of things as they are, combined with being prepared to work to improve the situation. For patients and their families, realism helps to avoid the depressive effect of negative rumination, which can lead to catastrophising, whilst deterring disappointment which may occur through unrealistic hopes of avoiding facing the true situation.

Shared decision-making focuses on including patients and their families in all decisions about their own lives so that their voices are heard, and their individual preferences understood and fully represented in any decision-making process which takes place.

Therapeutic silence allows time, space and capacity for cognitive patients to process and respond to information that has been provided. Silence can offer valuable thinking time for changing perspective and should be welcomed as an opportunity to support the person and reflect on the preceding interaction.

Whole person care involves responding to the needs and strengths of the whole person, including influences on their physical, social, psychological, and spiritual well-being, both now and in the past, whilst embedding the principles of person-centred care into every intervention.

MODELS

Chaplaincy in hospitals, hospices, and community settings often provides a diverse range of listening, support, and information services around matters to do with finding meaning, purpose, and understanding for patients with or without specific faith-based beliefs and traditions. As such, chaplains can contribute significant ways to the emotional and spiritual well-being of patients and their families as they adjust to loss and change.

Communities of believers are attributed different names within different faith-based traditions, including the following: congregations, assemblies, members, and brethren, to name only a few. What many communities of believers across a variety of faiths have in common is an understanding of the existence of a spiritual bond or relationship within and between the group of people making up the local, national and sometimes worldwide community.

Multi-faith chaplaincy is often the approach taken to providing hospital chaplaincy, although the actual range of faiths represented amongst the paid and voluntary chaplains will vary depending on and reflecting demographics in different localities. However, all multi-faith chaplaincies are likely to have contacts with ministers of religion from minority faiths in every local area. It can be particularly important for some people that rites and rituals towards or at the end of life are carried out by a person from their specific denomination rather than from a faith group which others consider to be similar.

References

Ali, M. (2018) Communication Skills 5: Effective listening and observation. *Nursing Times* [online]. 114(4): 56–57.

Antunes, M., Laranjeira, C., Querido, A. and Charepe, Z. (2023) "What Do We Know about Hope in Nursing Care?": A Synthesis of Concept Analysis Studies. *Healthcare* (Basel). 11(20): 2739. doi: 10.3390/healthcare11202739. PMID: 37893813; PMCID: PMC10606526.

DeForest, A. and Douglas, S.B. (2024) Total Pain: Euphemism and Mission Drift in the Treatment of Non-Physical Pain. *Journal of Pain and Symptom Management*. 67(5): e753–e754.

Department of Health (2012) *Compassion in Practice; Nursing, Midwifery and Care Staff; Our Vision and Strategy*. London: Gateway reference 18479.

Kubler-Ross, E. and Kessler, D. (2014) *On Grief & Grieving: Finding the Meaning of Grief through the Five Stages of Loss*. London: Simon and Schuster.

Nibbelink, C.W. and Brewer, B.B. (2018) Decision-Making in Nursing Practice: An Integrative Literature Review. *Journal of Clinical Nursing*. 27(5–6): 917–928.

Stenhouse, R. (2021) Understanding Equality and Diversity in Nursing Practice. *Nursing Standard* (Royal College of Nursing, Great Britain). 36(2): 27–33. https://doi.org/10.7748/ns.2020.e11562.

Case study 17
Zach: my choice, my voice

Kirsty Henry and Christine Nightingale

Meeting Zach

'We are not trained for this,' says Josie as she answers the door to me. Zach is my fifth visit this morning, and I am already running late. I introduce myself to Josie, trying to appear reassuring whilst experiencing the familiar feeling of dread, as I know that the conversation that we are about to have may be difficult. 'Please come in,' she says as she ushers me down the corridor to meet Zach in a small bedroom on the left-hand side.

'Hello Zach, my name is Jett, and I am a district nurse. Is it okay if I come in?' I say to him as I enter the room. Zach just grunts, but a woman sitting on a chair beside him states, 'Hello I'm Mary, Zach's mum, thanks for coming.'

APPROACH: "Hello my name is... campaign

Zach has recently been referred to us in the community nursing team for palliative care by the oncology team at the local hospital. I was keen to meet him as soon as possible, as he has an intellectual disability and Angelman Syndrome. In preparation for my visit, I took the opportunity to read about Angelman Syndrome, which I understand to be a rare genetic disorder which causes physical and cognitive disability. I learned that although symptoms vary for each individual, people with Angelman Syndrome often have a severe learning disability, and communication is frequently impaired. Therefore, I am not sure to what extent Zach understands the significance of his new diagnosis of Stage 4 colorectal cancer. Furthermore, I learned that gait disorders, gastric disorders, and epilepsy are common comorbidities of Angelman Syndrome, so I wonder if these comorbidities may impact upon Zach's presentation and whether the prevalence of gastrointestinal disorders has placed him at a higher risk of developing colorectal cancer. I have also read about common facial features in Angelman Syndrome, including a 'wide smile,' making me apprehensive of potentially misreading communication cues if

VALUE: curiosity

THEORY: Angelman syndrome

DOI: 10.4324/9781003651758-17

Zach uses facial expression to express his needs (Williams et al., 2010).

On entering Zach's room, I want to start building a relationship with him, as well as with his mother Mary and his carer Josie. I am conscious that there is potential for a lot of emotion within the room, alongside a number of questions to which I might not know the answers. The best place to begin to build my therapeutic relationship with them all is by finding out what they already know and what their worries are.

I walk towards Zach, ensuring that he can see me in the bedroom light, and I reach out to greet him by shaking his hand. Zach responds warmly with a smile, taking my hand, but I can see that his face grimaces from time to time. Although Zach does not use words to communicate, it is clear to me that he is able to express himself through body language. I wonder whether Josie and Mary use any additional methods to communicate with Zach. 'How do you know when Zach is in pain?' I ask. 'You can see it in his eyes,' Mary responds, bursting into tears.

Space to talk

Worried that seeing his mother upset might distress Zach, I suggest that we find somewhere else to talk. Eagerly, Josie agrees and directs us to an even smaller room off the entrance hall, which I can now see is the staff office.

As soon as we are in the quiet of the office, Mary says, 'I am so sorry, I just can't help worrying about what is going to happen. I don't want him to know that he's dying. He wouldn't understand, and it won't help him to know'. She goes on to explain: 'Everything is happening so fast, one minute he had a tummy ache, the next he's dying. They say he's too advanced, they can't treat him, and he wouldn't tolerate the treatment anyway'.

'It's not just that' Josie chips in 'we are a residential care home; we are not set up for end-of-life care.' She explains that Zach is a well-liked resident who has lived in the home for the past 15 years. 'He came to them as a young man of 30, straight from his parents' home, when things became too challenging for his family to manage. When Zach first moved in, he had frequent episodes of self-injurious behaviour. Over time we gained a good understanding of the triggers to his distress and through the introduction of new augmentative communication strategies we were able to support him and reduce his feelings of stress. From this, his ability to make decisions about his day to day needs and wishes using pictures and objects of reference, has developed.' Josie speaks warmly of Zach, going on to tell me that until recently he was happy and independently mobile; he could dress himself, take himself to the toilet, and feed himself.

> MODEL: self-injurious behaviours

> APPROACH: augmentative and alternative communication

> THEORY: informed choice

'Then, about 3 months ago, everything changed. He became withdrawn, spending more and more time on his own in his bedroom, usually lying on his bed. He went off his food, and when staff tried to help him, he would push them away' explains Josie.

> THEORY: atypical pain presentation

'We took him to the doctors, but they couldn't find anything wrong with him. They told us that bowel problems were common in Angelman Syndrome, and that he was just constipated. Zach wasn't in the mood to be examined, and there was no way they were going to be able to do anything more invasive. So, they just told us to keep an eye on him. We all thought he was just having an 'off moment.' And we weren't really sure what we were meant to be keeping an eye on.'

Josie looks at Mary as she says, 'He just got grumpier and grumpier; wouldn't let anyone near him. We all just thought that this was normal behaviour for someone with an intellectual disability. It wasn't until we noticed that his trousers were getting loose on him that we went back to the doctors, who then referred him to the hospital for tests. And now, here we are.

> THEORY: diagnostic overshadowing

More time to hear Zach's voice

I am conscious that I am already behind with my visits, and I want to begin to build a plan with Zach at the centre of it. I feel internally conflicted by the emotions and fears Josie and Mary have expressed, which could impact my care planning and assessment of his future needs. I am also mindful that there are potential commissioning challenges, as specialist interventions will have funding implications, and therefore, it may not be possible to provide optimal end-of-life care within his current residential care provision. Taking a deep breath, I suggest that we focus on Zach's immediate needs for now, explaining that I will come back again to talk about care options. I know that it is going to take several visits to get to know Zach, to be able to explore his preferences and to assess his capacity before I can even begin to establish which avenue may be the best to find the most appropriate care environment.

THEORY: Mental Capacity Act (2005)

APPROACH: best interests

'Hello Zach, it's me again, Jett - the district nurse. I've just been talking to your mum and Josie about helping to get rid of that pain. How does that sound?'

Zach smiles, but maybe that's just the Angelman Syndrome.

Reflections

This case stayed with me for the rest of the week. There were so many elements that caused me personal conflict and moral distress. My son is of a similar age, and therefore as a parent, I cannot help but consider whether things may have been different for Zach if he had had the range of life choices that my son has had. If Zach did not have an intellectual disability, I wonder whether his cancer might have been identified earlier, whether it might have been possible to offer him treatment, and whether he might be facing a more positive outcome.

The Learning from Lives and Deaths review body (LeDeR) aims to reduce the premature deaths of people with an intellectual disability and autistic people by reporting, annually, on the health inequalities experienced by this population in England. The average age at death for people with an intellectual disability is at least 20 years younger than the general population (White et al., 2023), with cancer repeatedly reported as one of the leading causes of death (Heslop et al., 2022; White et al., 2023). Although this is reported to correlate with people with an intellectual disability living longer, cancer, and colorectal cancer in particular, has been reported to disproportionally affect people with an intellectual disability, leading to death at an earlier age (Willis et al., 2018; Heslop et al., 2022; White et al., 2024). Late-stage reporting and referral is a significant contributing factor to premature mortality from colorectal cancer, alongside dietary intake and mobility limitations (White et al., 2024). I wonder whether these might have been contributing to Zach's case. I am not sure how easy it would have been for him to communicate the changes he was experiencing or, indeed, whether it is reasonable to expect those around him to have been able to recognise these changes and act upon them.

These thoughts lead me to consider the impact of Zach's non-verbal communication, both in relation to articulating his pain and other needs, and in relation to his decision-making. These have a significant impact on whether he has been empowered to engage with and make health-related decisions.

I am mindful that stage 4 cancer can be a painful condition, and it is vital that I support the carers and Mary to be able to recognise and monitor both the physical and emotional pain that Zach is likely to experience so that we can keep on top of this in his palliative care plan (Millard and de Knegt, 2019). People with an intellectual disability may express pain differently from people in the general population and would therefore suggest the adoption of the Disability Distress Assessment Tool (DisDAT) (St Oswald's Hospice and Northumberland Tyne and Wear NHS Trust, 2024) to help monitor his unique presentation. The DiSDAT is a validated tool which can help caregivers to recognise, record, and monitor the way that people express their pain, distress, and discomfort (Regnard et al., 2007).

It also troubled me that Zach's carer Josie was clearly concerned about her team's skill and the availability of resources to support Zach as his condition, progresses towards the end of life. It is not unusual for caregivers to be apprehensive over their capability and suitability to provide end-of-life care, but this may be compounded by Zach's intellectual disability. However, despite people with intellectual disabilities having a higher mortality rate than the general population, death is a rare experience within residential care settings for people with intellectual disabilities (Todd et al., 2019; Todd et al., 2020). Care provision for this population may differ from the care services established for a general population in that care may be long-term and more focused upon social needs than health needs. Zach's care team are not registered nurses, and they are not being funded to provide nursing care. Furthermore, Todd et al. (2020) highlight that death from cancer, which they describe as a condition traditionally associated with end-of-life care, relates to less than 20% of all deaths in intellectual disability settings. It is not surprising that staff working in a setting that has been a long-term provider of residential care for Zach have apprehensions over how they too can adjust to his changing needs and declining health. As a palliative care nurse, it is therefore important to support the care provider alongside Zach and his family.

During this first visit, valuable time was spent with Zach's mother Mary, as well as getting to know Zach's core care team within the service. This relationship-building is essential in ensuring that optimal support networks can be put in place as his health declines. These early conversations are an important part of my holistic nursing assessment, which will inform a flexible palliative care pathway for Zach. Speaking to Zach's family and care team will help me to establish Zach's wishes and preferences, which will in turn help with identifying which options may or may not be in his 'Best Interests' under the Mental Capacity Act (2005).

I am aware of some conflict with my core nursing values in person-centred practice. Zach's voice needs to remain at the centre of all my decision-making, and it is entirely possible that Zach would express a desire to remain in his current home, a place where he has lived for 15 years, and with carers who know him well. As a nurse, I need to ensure that I act as a professional advocate for his needs and his wishes (NMC, 2018). I wonder if I should have spent more time with Zach, as only by spending time with him will I begin to understand his communication methods and ensure that I can empower him to make his own choices. Although, in working with people that know him well, I can ensure that I can take a wider perspective when planning for his care. In England, the Mental Capacity Act (2005) clarifies that where a person lacks the capacity to make an informed decision, all reasonable steps must be taken to ensure that the person's wishes are considered as part of deciding what action is in their 'best interests'. I also need to consider what would be the 'least restrictive option.' Zach's carers and Mary can help me in these decision-making processes.

Central to his management are the issues of inclusion and informed consent. Mary has asked us not to tell Zach that he is dying. This is understandable but sits uncomfortably with a health practitioner's integrity. I wonder whether a lack of the whole truth is equivalent to a lie, and how I can work to empower Zach to make informed decisions if he does not know or understand what is happening to him. Indeed, how can I help him to understand and manage his symptoms if he does not know what is causing them or that they are likely to deteriorate. The tension between 'empowerment' and 'protection' risks unintended consequences of disempowerment, as well as adjustment difficulties for Zach which may impede his ability to provide consent. Truth-telling in palliative care with people with an intellectual disability is a complex area of practice (Cithambaram et al., 2020; Rauf and Bashir, 2021). A wrong step here could impede my relationship with Zach, his family, or his carers. Clearly, this is a subject to continue to reflect upon and to revisit in discussions with family and other professionals in Zach's care. It is important that we work together in a coherent way to ensure the best possible care for Zach and for his family and carers.

I will be making a referral to the Community Learning Disability Nurses for their specialist support to help address some of the issues identified in my reflection.

Questions for reflection and discussion

Explore the key issues raised in the above scenario as you answer the following six questions:

1. Identify at least six ways that Zach might communicate his needs and wishes.

2. Why is it important to challenge assumptions made about the health and care needs of people with an intellectual disability?

3. How might you involve someone with an intellectual disability in their own end-of-life care planning? What information do you need to seek from carers/family?

4. From which other health and social care professionals might you seek support in Zach's case, and how might they contribute to the decision-making processes?

5. What might be the challenges in seeking multiple viewpoints when working with a person who is unable to communicate verbally at the end of their life? How might you manage conflicting opinions?

6. Identify the arguments for and against informing Zach of his prognosis. Would you inform him? Explain the processes involved in making this decision.

Further reading

Hollins, S. and Tuffey-Wijne, I. (2018) *Am I going to Die?* Books Beyond Words. Available at: https://booksbeyondwords.co.uk/.

Mizen, L. (2024) Intellectual disability. *Medicine*, 52(8): 506–511, Available at: https://doi.org/10.1016/j.mpmed.2024.05.012.

Moore, C., Pan, C., Roseman, K., Stephens, M., Bien-Aime, C., Morgan, A., Ross, W., Castillo, M., Palathra, B., Jones, C., Ailey, S., Tuffrey-Wijne, I., Smeltzer, S. and Tobias, J. (2022) Top ten tips palliative care clinicians should know about navigating the needs of adults with intellectual disabilities. *Journal of Palliative Medicine*, 25(12): 1857–1864. Available at: https://doi.org/10.1089/jpm.2022.0384.

Tuffrey-Wijne, I. (2017) *A Life and Death Decision*. Available at: https://www.tuffrey-wijne.com.

Tuffrey-Wijne, I. and Willson, J. (2020) *Death and Dying* In: Heslop, P and Hebron, C (Eds) *Promoting the Health and Well-Being of People with Learning Disabilities*. Springer International Publishing. Available at: https://doi.org/10.1007/978-3-030-43488-5_8.

Further information

VALUES

Curiosity: Professional curiosity enables practitioners to proactively assess, analyse, and understand a presenting situation. Being curious enables an enhanced exploration of risk, helps to build a respectful therapeutic relationship and creates a culture of learning through preparation and reflection.

Truth-telling: Decisions on whether, how much, and how to communicate with people with intellectual disabilities about their own mortality are becoming increasingly important for healthcare services. Historically, only half of people with intellectual disabilities who were terminally ill were informed about their illness, and less than 20% were told they would die. Irene Tuffrey-Wijne has written extensively on breaking bad news for people with an intellectual disability.

THEORIES

Angelman syndrome is a rare genetic neurodevelopmental condition causing physical and intellectual disability. Signs and symptoms can vary widely among individuals but usually become apparent in infancy and are lifelong. Associated characteristics include developmental delay, including limited verbal communication skills, movement disorders, microcephaly, scoliosis, and distinct facial features, including a wide mouth and pale skin and hair colour. People with Angelman Syndrome often experience gastric disorders including constipation and reflux, and epilepsy is common in this population. Behavioural traits include hyperactivity, frequent episodes of laughter, flapping of hands, anxiety, sleep disorders, and episodes of self-injurious behaviour.

Atypical pain presentation is an umbrella term which is used to capture non-characteristic presentations of pain. Signs and symptoms may be subtle in people with intellectual disabilities and therefore it is important to observe and report changes in behaviour and body language in addition to explicit expressions of pain. The DisDAT tool (Regnard et al., 2007) may be helpful in identifying and recording atypical pain presentations.

Diagnostic overshadowing occurs when clinicians make assumptions based on a person's underlying condition. People with an intellectual disability may have challenges in recognising and/or communicating a health need and are often reliant upon others to identify the need and take appropriate action. This can result in symptoms being overlooked, particularly when they are attributed to the underlying condition or intellectual disability. For example, the facial features and behavioural traits seen in Angelman Syndrome can lead to assumptions made in relation to an absence of pain and discomfort.

Informed choice for a person to consent to treatment or a procedure, or to deny consent, they must be given all the information about that treatment or procedure, including potential benefits, side effects, alternatives, and consequences of not undergoing treatment. However, it is not sufficient to simply provide information; clinicians must ensure that the information is accessible to the person to enable them to make an informed decision. This may involve adjustments to language, settings, text information, or the use of alternative formats, including Easy Read information. The NHS Accessible Information Standards (NHS England, 2017) provide statutory guidance to help you explore the sharing of information which is accessible to enable informed choice.

Mental Capacity Act (2005) provides a legislative framework to support decision-making for people aged 16 and over in England and Wales. It establishes five principles, including the presumption of capacity, clarifies a four-stage test to assess capacity, and provides a clear process of decision-making when a person is assessed to lack the capacity to make a specific decision.

Non-verbal communication is a term used to describe any form of communication that is used excluding spoken language or words.

Unconscious bias in learning disability care: clinical decisions are made with the best of intentions, based on knowledge, skill, and experience; however, it is important to be aware of one's unconscious biases. In Learning Disability Practice, decisions can be influenced by a perceived inability to cope with or consent to treatment or by assumptions about a person's quality of life (Tuffrey-Wijne et al., 2013; White et al., 2023).

APPROACHES

Augmentative and alternative communication (AAC) incorporates a wide range of techniques that support (*augment*) or *replace* spoken communication. These include 'no-tech' means such as gestures, body language, and sign-language, 'low-tech' means such as objects of reference and pictures, such as Easy Read and 'high tech' means including tablets, electronic communication boards and Voice Output Communication Aids (VOCAs). AACs enable communication to be as effective as possible.

Best interests is the process of determining the outcome of the decision is in a person's best interests in the event that they are assessed as lacking the capacity to make that decision under the Mental Capacity Act (2005).

"Hello my name is..." campaign is an approach founded by Dr Kate Granger prior to her death in 2016. As a patient with terminal cancer, Kate identified what she described as a 'stark reality' that clinicians were failing to introduce themselves before delivering care. As a clinician, Kate understood the importance of communication in the delivery of compassionate healthcare. #Hellomynameis has four key values: Communication, The Little Things, Patients at the Heart of all Decisions and See me. For more information on Kate's campaign and legacy alongside these core values can be found at https://www.hellomynameis.org.uk/.

Involving and supporting family and carers in palliative care is not just for the person who is ill but for all the people who are important in their life. People with an intellectual disability may have different social networks than those in the general population, including close relationships with parents, siblings, friends, and carers. It is important to establish who is important to that person and ensure that they are involved as partners in care and offered support.

Relationship building: The NMC Code (2018) requires all registered nurses to act in partnership with those receiving care, helping them to access relevant health and social care, information and support when they need it.

MODELS

Reflection in action is a process by which practitioners analyse practice, thoughts, feelings, and values as they go about their work.

Self-injurious behaviour is a behaviour that a person engages in which causes physical harm to themselves. Self-injurious behaviour can vary in intensity and has potential to be dangerous, and can therefore be challenging to observe. Although this behaviour is not uncommon in working with people with intellectual disabilities, the causes are complex, and referral for support from specialist services is recommended. Self-injurious behaviour is different from self-harm, which is deliberate in nature.

References

Cithambaram, K., Duffy, M. and Courtney, E. (2020) Disclosure and plan of care at end of life: Perspectives of people with intellectual disabilities and families in Ireland. *British Journal of Learning Disabilities*, 48(4): 340–347.

Heslop, P., Cook, A., Sullivan, B., Calkin, R., Pollard, J. and Byrne, V. (2022) Cancer in deceased adults with intellectual disabilities: English population-based study using linked data from three sources. *British Medical Journal Open*, 12(3): e056974. Available at: https://doi.org/10.1136/bmjopen-2021-056974.

Mental Capacity Act (MCA) 2005, c. 9. Available at: https://www.legislation.gov.uk/ukpga/2005/9/contents/enacted (Accessed 31st January 2025).

Millard, S. and de Knegt, N. (2019) Cancer pain in people with intellectual disabilities: Systematic review and survey of health care professionals. *Journal of Pain and Symptom Management*, 58(6): 1081–1099.

NHS England (2017) Accessible Information Standard Implementation Guidance v1.1. Available at: https://www.england.nhs.uk/publication/accessible-information-standard-implementation-guidance/

Nursing and Midwifery Council (2018) *The Code: Professional Standards of Practice and Behaviour for Nurses, Midwives and Nursing Associates*. NMC, London.

Rauf, L. and Bashir, K (2021) Challenges of providing palliative care to a patient with learning disability: A case study from United Kingdom General Practice. *Cureus*, 13(4): E14240.

Regnard, C., Reynolds, J., Watson, B., Matthews, D., Gibson, L. and Clarke, C. (2007) Understanding distress in people with severe communication difficulties: Developing and assessing the Disability Distress Assessment Tool (DisDAT). *Journal of Intellectual Disability Research*, 51(4): 277–292.

Todd, S., Bernal, J., Shearn, J., Worth, R., Jones, E., Lowe, K., Madden, P., Barr, O., Forrester Jones, R., Jarvis, P., Kroll, T., McCarron, M., Read, S. and Hunt, K. (2020) Last months of life of people with intellectual disabilities: A UK population-based study of death and dying in intellectual disability community services. *Journal of Applied Research in Intellectual Disabilities*, 33(6): 1245–1258.

St Oswald's Hospice and Northumberland Tyne and Wear NHS Trust (2024) Distress and Discomfort Assessment Tool (DisDAT v22). Available at: https://www.stoswaldsuk.org/wp-content/uploads/2024/10/disdat-22-Web.pdf (Accessed 31st January 2025).

Todd, S., Brandford, S., Worth, R., Shearn, J. and Bernal, J. (2019) Place of death of people with intellectual disabilities: An exploratory study of death and dying within community disability service settings. *Journal of Intellectual Disability*, 33: 1245–1258. Available at: https://doi.org/10.1177/1744629519886758.

Tuffrey-Wijne, I., Giatras, N., Goulding, L., Abraham, E., Fenwick, L., Edwards, C. and Hollins, S. (2013) Identifying the factors affecting the implementation of strategies to promote a safer environment for patients with learning disabilities in NHS hospitals: A mixed-methods study. *Health Services and Delivery Research*, 1(13): 1–224. Available at: https://doi.org/10.3310/hsdr01130.

White, A., Sheehan, R., Ding, J., Roberts, C., Magill, N., Keagan-Bull, R., Carter, B. and Strydom, A. (2023) *Learning from Lives and Deaths – People with a learning disability and autistic people* (LeDeR) report for 2022. London, UK.

White, A., Roberts, C., Ding, J., Sheehan, R., Sanger, E., Chauhan, U. and Strydom, A. (2024) Bowel cancer in people with a learning disability: An international comparison and discussion of lowering the age of screening based on LeDeR data. Kings Colledge London. Available at: https://www.kcl.ac.uk/ioppn/leder/bowel-cancer-deep-dive.pdf (Accessed 31st January 2025).

Williams, C.A., Driscoll, D.J. and Dagli, A.I. (2010) Clinical and genetic aspects of Angelman syndrome. *Genetics in Medicine*, 12(7): 385–395. Available at: https://doi.org/10.1097/GIM.0b013e3181def138.

Willis, D., Samalin, E. and Satgé, D. (2018) Colorectal cancer in people with intellectual disabilities. *Oncology*, 95(6): 323–336. Available at: https://doi.org/10.1159/000492077.

Case study 18
Joan: should I stay or should I go now?

Simon Rose

The case in question

Should I stay or should I go now? Yes, it's a reference to an iconic punk rock song, but also the key question that every out-of-hospital paramedic needs to ask themselves at the end of their consultations. Working as a specialist paramedic in primary and urgent care gives no exemptions from this question. Although I have advanced training that permits me to carry more medications in my arsenal of treatment options, the fundamental question remains... should this patient stay at home? Can they be safely managed in the community, or do they need to go to the hospital for additional treatment and management that cannot be accessed in the community? The question appears simple, but the journey to the answer can be complex, multifaceted, and dynamic. Imagine trying to catch moving pieces of a puzzle before you even know what the picture of the puzzle looks like. Clinical decision-making is complicated, and Joan's case breaks down some of the complexity around the decision-making process, slowing down the moving pieces of the puzzle presented.

From call to arrival

Joan is a 76-year-old female referred to the emergency services via the 111 service. As a specialist paramedic, I have been asked to attend the call. The drive to Joan's house is only a few miles, but I take the opportunity to wonder what may await me upon my arrival. One of the common pitfalls with emergency calls is that the information given at the time of the call is often only the tip of the iceberg, and presentations can often vary significantly from what they first appear to be. I am aware it is one of the first opportunities for different forms of potential cognitive biases, such as anchoring bias, to creep into the thought

VALUE: curiosity

THEORY: anchoring bias

DOI: 10.4324/9781003651758-18

VALUE: self-awareness

process of any clinician. I pull up to the bungalow for the address given, and although it is dark, I can instantly see a pristine front garden, one that is clearly kept with real pride. With my kit bag on and my hands full of devices, I approach the front door and am instantly greeted by a man who takes me through to the lounge area of the property. This is where I meet Joan, who is semi-recumbent in a hospital bed, which is often a sign of reduced mobility and

MODEL: global overview

deteriorating health. In my experience, a hospital bed in the home is normally there out of necessity rather than an interior design choice.

Initiating the consultation and gathering Information

APPROACH: "Hello, my name is ..." campaign

APPROACH: communication

I initiate the consultation by introducing myself, highlighting my role and asking the names of both the gentlemen in the room and the lady in bed in front of me. I confirm Joan is my patient, and the gentleman with her is John, her husband. I invite Joan to outline her primary complaint in her own words to reduce any potential bias that may be

THEORY: anchoring bias

lingering from the call information I have received prior to

VALUE: respect

my arrival. I make sure not to interject, as interruptions of

APPROACH: golden minute

a patient's opening dialogue have been found to be detrimental to clinical outcomes. At the same time, I adopt an open and receptive style of body language to show Joan

APPROACH: active listening

I am actively listening to what she is saying. I am aware non-verbal techniques, such as using appropriate body

THEORY: non-verbal communication

movement, facial expressions, eye contact and showing interest in the patient's words, all contribute to successful

APPROACH: building patient rapport

rapport building with a patient.

The information I gather is as much from John as from Joan, with the opening dialogue being like a double act. Joan starts a sentence, and John finishes it. I wonder whether this could be a theme within their relationship as husband and wife, or whether it might be a behaviour change due to the stress of the situation. Nevertheless, it

THEORY: social complexity

adds a level of social complexity. Joan looks tired but still

APPROACH: observational assessment

responds verbally to me when I ask a question. From our opening exchanges, I establish that Joan is a retired nurse, living with her husband, John. Joan has been diagnosed with lung cancer, which is compounded by her existing chronic obstructive pulmonary disease (COPD) that she has lived with for several years. One observation that is very clear is that Joan has a supportive home environment with John, who is now her primary caregiver. He appears keen to make sure her every need is attended to.

John expresses concern that Joan was relatively stable until her last round of chemotherapy, around four weeks ago. I am keen to explore her signs and symptoms further by asking what has changed over the past few weeks. Joan appears embarrassed but replies, 'I am sleeping for large parts of the day and can't walk more than a few steps so can't ever get to the toilet in time.' John adds that her colour is pale compared to her usual complexion and that she has not been able to get out of bed for the past few days. I enquire how her breathing is compared to her normal baseline of breathlessness, and she replies with a sense of irony. 'To be honest that is only thing that has not really changed, in fact I now cough less!' As we discuss the history of her presenting complaint, it becomes clear that, as a retired nurse, Joan has a good level of understanding of clinical conditions and of the process she is going through medically, psychologically, and socially. At this point, I catch myself thinking that today she may be the patient, but she has stood in my shoes at the bedside of many patients over the course of her career, and it must be hard for her to be on the other side.

I continue to gain a history from Joan by investigating her medical and social history with further open questions. Joan highlights that up until her retirement 10 years ago, she had no medical issues. 'However,' her tone of voice changes as she states with a guilty but bashful look on her face, 'I have been a smoker since I was a teenager.' I know the look well, as it is the same look I see when I catch one of my children doing something they know they should not be doing. 'The years of smoking have finally caught up with me,' she adds. Joan talks about how she knew she had COPD soon after retiring. 'I had seen it all before, the

APPROACH: functional inquiry

VALUE: curiosity

APPROACH: empathy

MODEL: Calgary Cambridge Model of Consultation

THEORY: open questioning

VALUE: acceptance

breathlessness, fatigue and that awful hacking cough. Her tone darkens further as she highlights that over the past 10 years her health has just declined year on year. 'I've lost count of how many antibiotic courses I've had since I was diagnosed with COPD and then last year, I started to get pain in my chest and that's when they found the lung cancer.' I ask how long Joan has been living with cancer, to which she smirks, saying, 'This does not feel like living.' I get the sense that Joan is resigned to the fact her health is on a downward spiral.

John was much more positive and jumped into the conversation to add that they were due to see the oncology consultant in a couple of weeks to discuss how Joan had responded to the latest round of chemotherapy. He continued by adding that she was sometimes confused, stating, 'Since she finished her last round of chemotherapy, she has not been herself.' His expression changes slightly as he now looks bemused, 'She walked into the hospital that day and has barely walked since.' There is an element of stress in his voice, as though he has run out

APPROACH: compassionate communication

VALUE: caring

of ideas of how he can support Joan. I move to reassure John, acknowledging what a difficult period this must be for both of them.

I take the opportunity to explore the social aspects of the situation more. 'So, John, do you have any support for you or Joan at all?' John looks slightly puzzled by the question, so I refine it further, asking 'Do you have any carers come in to give you a hand with Joan? Help with getting her washed and dressed for example?' John is almost defiant in his response, saying 'No, no, no. I do not need help to look after my wife. I assure John that he is doing a great job, while also highlighting that if he is struggling, support can be arranged for both Joan and him. I conclude my information gathering by exploring what healthcare input they have had recently. John explains that they have not seen anyone since the last round of chemotherapy four weeks ago, but prior to that had been visited by a nurse from the palliative care team, who had helped them organise the hospital bed and given them a folder of paperwork.

APPROACH: situational communication styles

THEORY: caregiver burnout

The last part of that sentence made my ears perk up. As a paramedic, I know that the palliative care pack could either be my best friend or worst enemy in terms of making clinical decisions regarding patients with cancer. A pack that has been filled out comprehensively with the patient's wishes, a respect form, or an advanced care directive can not only support but really guide a clinician towards the best possible outcome for a patient. However, a pack that includes vague or mixed messages regarding the patient's wishes can be damaging to the patient, not only in the current context of this case but in future situations. It could even impact the patient's ability to have a 'good death' on their own terms in some cases. A report of a recent patient consultation instantly comes to my mind, which unfortunately had a pack that was completely blank and left the patient exposed to receiving treatment against their wishes. Although heuristic at this point is automatic, it is vital to have this awareness of potential bias. As clinicians, we should not automatically lock on To individual pieces of information that may influence the judgement of the consultation. I task John with finding the pack for me so we can review it together. This also buys me some time to complete a physical examination of Joan.

MODEL: gold standard palliative framework

THEORY: availability bias

APPROACH: information gathering

Physical examination

I start the examination by explaining what I am going to do and gaining Joan's consent. I then review her appearance, having already made a mental note that John referred to her complexion as being 'pale' compared to usual, and although I am not aware of Joan's normal complexion, it is evident she lacks warmth in her skin tone but also has no cyanotic features. Joan knows the routine well, probably having done it thousands of times herself, but it further allows me to establish some of the key pieces of the puzzle that I am starting to put together.

APPROACH: informed consent

APPROACH: end of bed assessment

Joan's pulse is 104 beats per minute at rest, she has a respiratory rate of 24, oxygenation saturation of 90%, and her blood pressure is 94/56. 'Do you feel feverish, Joan?' I ask, to which she replies, 'Yes, at times'. I use my tympanic thermometer to take her temperature, which, to my surprise, flashes up as 37.5 degrees. I was expecting it to be higher given Joan's comments about feeling feverish and her presentation with features of a potential underlying infection. I resist the temptation to seek out further findings that purely supported this thought process and complete some more focused assessments, including a respiratory examination and a functional test of her motor functions. Joan's lung sounds identify some fine bilateral crackles to her lower right base, which may indicate pathology from an underlying infection, but could also be a normal finding for a patient with COPD. The functional assessment highlights that although she is very weak, she can perform fine and gross motor movements of all four limbs, although no weight-bearing assessment is completed at this stage. At this point John returns with the documentation left by the palliative care nurse.

THEORY: confirmation bias

Explanation and planning

With John now back in the room, I start to summarise my clinical findings to both of them, including explaining how Joan's presentation links to her history and presenting symptoms. Joan's blood pressure is a concern to me, and the raised temperature and heart rate might be signs of an infective pathophysiology, although no singular source stands out. The noted urinary incontinence could be a sign of a urinary tract infection, but with no other symptoms reported, it is far from a clear diagnosis. I also raise my concern about the deterioration from mobile to immobile since her last chemotherapy along with the fact that no healthcare assessment or follow-up has been completed over this time. I continue to explain that as Joan is actively having chemotherapy, this increases her risk of neutropenia and potentially neutropenic sepsis, which is treatable and could greatly improve Joan's symptoms.

THEORY: clinical reasoning

Before continuing the consultation by discussing the pathway options available to Joan and John, I review the palliative care folder that John has handed to me. My heart sinks slightly when I find page after page with empty sections. I ask John if anyone had gone through this folder with either of them to which he replies, 'Not really. The nurse gave us the folder and told us a bit about what it was for, but that was it.'

'Joan, based on my findings I think you require urgent hospital review. If you agree, I would like to book urgent ambulance transport to your local hospital.' Joan's expression changes to one of sadness, 'Do I really have to go in?' From a patient-centred perspective, Joan's wishes are hugely important and must be considered as part of an ethical decision-making framework. Before I can answer, John interjects, 'Joan, please get the treatment you need.' This was the first sign that John might be struggling at home with Joan's deterioration, and after an emotive discussion, the pair agree to my recommendation for hospitalisation.

> MODEL: ethical decision-making

Closing the consultation

As the main consultation naturally comes to its conclusion, I outline what will happen, and I request an ambulance for Joan. John instantly tasks himself with gathering an overnight bag, including any items Joan may need. I explain that due to operational pressures, the ambulance could be several hours. However, this time affords me the opportunity to talk to John and Joan about what her wishes are for her general health moving forward. We go over some of the questions within the palliative care pack and document how Joan and John would like to prioritise her care in the future, especially if she and John are in a situation where Joan may not be able to verbalise her decisions to a healthcare professional. These conversations can be difficult, and clinicians need to assess whether patients and their loved ones are ready to undertake such a discussion. However, when done correctly, such conversations lay the foundations to facilitate the patient to have a 'good death'. An hour after requesting ambulance transport, a double-staffed ambulance arrives to take Joan to the hospital. Therefore, to answer my introductory question of 'should I stay, or should I go now?' it was the latter.

> APPROACH: making every contact count

> VALUE: honesty

> THEORY: a good death

Reflections

Maintaining a patient-centred approach throughout the consultation process reminded me of the critical need to address not only the medical requirements but also emotional and psychological support for both Joan and John. Recognising that healthcare extends beyond physical ailments is vital, as patients often experience a myriad of feelings, including fear, anxiety, and uncertainty during their healthcare interactions. Providing holistic care that encompasses these aspects but fosters a more compassionate environment and strengthens the rapport between healthcare providers and patients.

The ethical complexities inherent in Joan's case necessitate careful navigation. Balancing Joan's autonomy with her pressing short-term health needs requires a nuanced understanding of her wishes and values. It was essential to engage in advanced care planning discussions even amidst the emotive experience of an unscheduled healthcare visit. Such conversations, though challenging, are imperative for ensuring that treatment strategies are not only clinically appropriate but also honour patients' desires and beliefs. This alignment not only respects patient autonomy but also promotes a sense of advocacy, which can be particularly empowering in difficult situations.

Joan's case serves as a poignant reminder of the intricate nature of out-of-hospital care within the context of acute-on-chronic presentations. It illustrates how healthcare providers must integrate theoretical frameworks, ethical principles, and a patient-centred ethos to navigate challenging scenarios effectively. The complexities of this case underscore the necessity of fostering resilience and adaptability among providers, as well as the importance of collaboration between patients and healthcare staff to ensure that all aspects of patient care are ethical and tailored to the individual.

Moreover, this experience reinforces the need for me to maintain ongoing education and training in managing complex medical situations. Continuous professional development ensures that healthcare teams are equipped with the knowledge and skills to respond adeptly, providing not only high-quality medical care but also emotional support during critical moments. It is a reminder that care must be tailored to the individual's unique context, promoting their dignity and enhancing their experience throughout the healthcare journey.

Through this experience, I gained invaluable insights into the paramount importance of compassionate communication. This involves actively listening to patients and their families, validating their feelings, and ensuring they feel heard and understood. Such communication fosters trust and can significantly impact the overall experience of care, promoting better health outcomes and patient satisfaction.

Questions for reflection and discussion

Explore the key issues raised in the above scenario as you answer the following six questions:

1. Within your current scope of practice, identify how you may have handled communication and decision-making in Joan's case.

2. If you were struggling to make a clinical decision, what support mechanisms do you have that could help you?

3. What additional clinical expertise may have been useful to access in this case?

4. What might some of the wider impact be on John if Joan had not been referred to the hospital for acute assessment and treatment?

5. Describe the benefits and risks of using a consultation model such as the Calgary Cambridge consultation model to assess a patient like Joan?

6. What types of cognitive bias (anchoring, availability, and confirmation) might impact you in your decision-making and why?

Further reading

Blackmore, T. (2022) *Palliative and end of life care for paramedics*, Bridgewater, Class Professional Publishing.

Collen, A. (2022) *Decision making in paramedic practice*, Bridgewater, Class Professional Publishing.

Edwards, A. (2009) *Shared decision-making in health care: Achieving evidence-based patient choice*, Oxford, Oxford University Press.

Pryde, N. (2022) *Enhanced palliative care: A handbook for paramedics, nurses and doctors*, Bridgewater, Class Professional Publishing.

Rutherford, G. (2022) *Human factors in paramedic practice*, Bridgewater, Class Professional Publishing.

Further information

VALUES

Acceptance is a core aspect of person-centred practice. It works together with being non-judgmental and understanding the individual's perspective, serving as a fundamental principle when working with people living with cancer throughout their journey. This approach is essential for promoting patient well-being.

Caring involves practitioners engaging in interactions and interventions that address the needs of the individual within their unique context. It also includes applying an evidence-based approach to ensure the right care is provided in a timely manner at every stage of life.

Curiosity goes beyond what meets the eye, through observing, listening, asking questions, and thinking critically about the information collected.

Honesty is an essential quality in any person working in healthcare, due to the vulnerability of service users many of whom will be living with long-term illnesses or conditions, which may make them fully or partially dependent on the care and support of others.

Respect involves recognising and acknowledging the unconditional value of all people.

Self-awareness in practitioners delivering health and care services is essential for reflective practice, providing person-centred care, and using oneself therapeutically to build relationships based on a shared understanding of what matters most to the patient.

THEORIES

Anchoring bias refers to the practice of prioritising information that supports one's initial impression of the information, even when those impressions are incorrect (Senay and Kaphlngst, 2008).

Availability bias is the tendency to overestimate the likelihood of events when they readily come to mind. For example, clinicians may recall a recent presentation and link it to a different patient even if the probability is minimal.

Caregiver burnout refers to the physical, emotional, and mental exhaustion that caregivers may experience after prolonged periods of providing care for a loved one, often due to the demands of their caregiving role. Caregivers, whether for family members with chronic illnesses, disabilities, or ageing-related issues, can become overwhelmed by the responsibilities they carry. Burnout can affect their own well-being, making it harder for them to continue providing effective care (Bevans and Sternburg, 2012).

Clinical reasoning refers to the process healthcare professionals use to gather, interpret, and analyse patient information to make informed decisions about diagnosis, treatment, and care. It involves the ability to think critically and systematically to assess patient conditions, recognise patterns, and determine the best course of action.

Confirmation bias involves selectively gathering information to conform with one's belief, as well as neglecting evidence that contradicts this belief. For example, refusing to consider an alternative diagnosis once an initial diagnosis has been made, even after testing may contradict it.

Good death refers to a death that aligns with the wishes and values of the person who is dying, ensuring comfort, dignity, and peace in their final moments. It is about creating an environment that supports the emotional, physical, social, and spiritual needs of the patient, and ideally, the family as well.

Non-verbal communication refers to the transmission of messages or information without using words. It includes body language, facial expressions, gestures, posture, eye contact, tone of voice, and even things like clothing or personal space. It is a huge part of how we communicate because it can convey emotions, attitudes, and reactions, sometimes even more strongly than words can. For example, a smile can express friendliness, while crossed arms might signal defensiveness (Fassaert et al., 2007).

Open questioning refers to the technique of asking questions that encourage expansive, thoughtful responses rather than simple "yes" or "no" answers. These types of questions are designed to stimulate conversation, critical thinking, and deeper exploration of ideas or issues. Open questions often begin with words like "how," "why," "what," or "tell me about," and they require more explanation or insight (Little et al., 2001).

Social complexity refers to the intricate web of relationships, roles, norms, and behaviours that exist within a society and how they may impact individuals. It highlights how individuals or groups interact with each other, and how various social structures, such as institutions, communities, and networks, shape and influence these interactions. The more diverse and interconnected the relationships and roles within a society, the greater its social complexity.

APPROACHES

Active listening is a communication technique where the listener fully concentrates, understands, responds, and remembers what the speaker is saying. It goes beyond just hearing words; it is about engaging with the speaker and making sure they feel heard and understood. In active listening, the listener is not just passively absorbing information but is actively involved in the conversation (Bryant, 2009).

Building patient rapport refers to creating a trusting, respectful, and empathetic relationship between a healthcare provider and a patient. It is about establishing a connection that makes the patient feel comfortable, valued, and understood, which in turn can improve communication and the overall healthcare experience (Jahromi et al., 2016).

Communication is central to successful caring relationships and to effective teamworking. Listening is as important as what we say and do.

Compassionate communication refers to the way healthcare providers interact with patients in a manner that is empathetic, respectful, and considerate of the patient's emotional, mental, and physical needs. It involves actively listening, showing understanding, and responding with kindness while addressing both the medical and emotional aspects of a patient's care (Edwards, 2009).

Empathy is essential for providing person-centred care. It enables the person providing support to better understand the world from the perspective of the patient, and therefore to respond to their experience of service delivery with an individualised approach (Jones, 2003).

End-of-bed assessment is a quick, informal evaluation of a patient's overall condition conducted by a healthcare provider while standing at the foot of the patient's bed. It is often used to gather an initial impression of a patient's health status. The goal is to rapidly assess key aspects of the patient's condition, such as their appearance, alertness, mobility, and any immediate signs of distress or complications, without having to perform a more detailed examination right away.

Functional inquiry refers to the process of asking questions to assess how a patient can perform daily activities and manage their overall functioning in life. It is a way for healthcare providers to gather information about the patient's physical, cognitive, and emotional abilities, and to identify any challenges or limitations they may be facing. This can help guide diagnosis, treatment, and rehabilitation plans.

Golden minute refers to the first minute of a healthcare consultation, which is seen as crucial in establishing a positive and trusting relationship between the healthcare provider and the patient. The concept is rooted in the idea that the way a healthcare professional begins the conversation can set the tone for the rest of the consultation (Dains et al., 2012).

"Hello, my name is …" campaign is an initiative that focuses on improving communication between healthcare providers and patients. It began in 2013 with Dr Kate Granger, a doctor who was diagnosed with terminal cancer. After her diagnosis, she realised that many healthcare professionals would often introduce themselves by their titles but rarely by their names. This lack of personal connection frustrated her, so she started the campaign to encourage healthcare workers to introduce themselves to patients by their first names, fostering more human-centred interactions and improving patient experiences.

Information gathering refers to the process of collecting relevant data about a patient's health, medical history, lifestyle, and current symptoms. This information helps healthcare providers make informed decisions, diagnose conditions, develop treatment plans, and provide appropriate care (Silverman et al., 2008).

Informed consent is a critical component in providing patient-centred care in healthcare settings. These processes ensure that patients are fully informed and agree to the care or procedures being performed.

Making every contact count is an approach that emphasises the importance of using every interaction with a patient or individual as an opportunity to promote health and well-being. This approach encourages healthcare providers to integrate health messages, advice, and support into all types of contacts, whether they are related to the specific reason for the visit or not.

Observational assessment is a method of gathering information about a patient's condition, behaviour, or responses by directly observing them, rather than relying solely on patient reports or diagnostic tests. Healthcare providers use this approach to assess various aspects of a patient's health, such as physical abilities, emotional state, cognitive function, or the effectiveness of a treatment plan.

Patient-centred care focuses on tailoring care to meet the unique needs, preferences, and values of the individual patient. It emphasises treating the patient as a whole person, rather than just addressing their medical condition, and involves engaging patients in their own care process (Sommer et al., 2016).

Situational communication style refers to the way a person adjusts their communication based on the context, audience, and situation they are in. In healthcare, this means adapting your tone, language, and approach depending on factors like the patient's condition, their emotional state, or the nature of the conversation. The goal is to ensure that the message is delivered effectively and appropriately, promoting understanding and positive interactions (Smith, 2004).

MODELS

Calgary-Cambridge model of consultation is a widely recognised framework used in medical practice to guide effective communication between healthcare professionals and patients (Harrison et al., 2007). The model outlines a structured approach to patient interviews, ensuring that important information is gathered, the patient feels heard, and both clinical and emotional aspects of care are addressed. It was developed by researchers at the University of Calgary and the University of Cambridge (Kurtz and Silverman, 1996).

Ethical decision-making is a framework designed to guide healthcare professionals through complex ethical dilemmas, helping them to make decisions that are well-reasoned, balanced, and aligned with ethical principles. The model provides a structured approach to analyse situations where ethical challenges arise, particularly when there may be conflicting values or interests. Ethical principles include:

- **Autonomy**: Respecting the patient's rights to make decisions about their own care.

- **Beneficence**: Acting in the best interest of the patient, promoting their well-being.

- **Non-maleficence**: Avoiding harm to the patient.

- **Justice**: Treating patients fairly and distributing resources equitably. These principles can help clarify the ethical implications of each option.

Global overview in patient assessment refers to a comprehensive, wide-ranging evaluation of the patient's overall condition, both at the scene of the emergency and during transport. It involves looking at the patient holistically, considering all factors that might impact their health and how different systems (physical, mental, and emotional) could be affected.

Gold standard framework for palliative care is often referred to as the gold standard framework (GSF). It is a structured model aimed at improving the care of patients in the last year of life, focusing on providing high-quality, coordinated, and compassionate care. This framework is widely used in various healthcare settings to guide the management of palliative patients, especially in primary care, but it can be applied in hospitals, hospices, and home care as well.

References

Bevans, M. and Sternberg, E. (2012) Caregiving burden, stress, and health effects among family caregivers of adult cancer patients. *Journal of the American Medical Association*, 307(4): 398–403. doi: 10.1001/jama.2012.29. PMID: 22274687; PMCID: PMC3304539.

Bryant, L. (2009) The art of active listening. *Practice Nurse*, 37(6): 49–52.

Dains, J., Baumann, L. and Scheibel, P. (2012) *Advanced Health Assessment and Clinical Diagnosis in Primary Care*. Mosby, St Louis.

Edwards, M. (2009) *Communication Skills for Nurses: A Practical Guide on How to Achieve Successful Consultations*. Andrews UK Ltd., Luton, Bedfordshire.

Fassaert, T., van Dulmen, S., Schellevis, F. and Bensing, J. (2007) Active listening in medical consultations: Development of the Active Listening Observation Scale (ALOS-global). *Patient Education and Counselling*, 68 (3): 258–264.

Harrison, C., Hart, J. and Wass, V. (2007) Learning to Communicate using the Calgary-Cambridge Framework. *Clinical Teacher*, 4(3): 159–164.

Jahromi, V., Tabatabaee, S., Adbar, Z. and Rajabi, M. (2016) Active listening: The key to successful communication in hospital managers. *Electron Physician,* 8(3): 2123–2128.

Jones, A. (2003) Nurses talking to patients: Exploring conversation analysis as a means of researching nurse-patient communication. *International Journal of Nursing Studies*, 40(6): 608–618.

Kurtz, S. and Silverman, J. (1996) The Calgary-Cambridge Referenced Observation Guides: An aid to defining the curriculum and organising the teaching in communication training programmes. *Med Education*, 30(2): 83–89.

Little, P., Everitt, H., Williamson, I., Warner, G., Moore, M., Gould, C., Ferrier, K. and Payne, S. (2001) Observational study of effect of patient centredness and positive approach on outcomes of general practice consultations. *British Medical Journal*, 323(7318): 908–911.

Senay, I. and Kaphingst, K. (2008) Anchoring and adjustment bias in communication of disease risk. *Society for Medical Decision Making*, 29(2): 193–201.

Silverman, J., Kurtz, S. and Draper, J. (2008) *Skills for Communicating with Patients*. Radcliffe Medical Press, Oxford.

Smith, S. (2004) Nurse practitioner consultations: Communicating with style and expertise. *Primary Health Care*, 14(10): 37–41.

Sommer, J., Lanier, C., Perron, N., Nendaz, M., Clavet, D. and Audétat, M. (2016) A teaching skills assessment tool inspired by the Calgary–Cambridge model and the patient-centred approach. *Patient Education and Counselling*, 99(4): 600–609.

Conclusion

We hope you found the case studies in this book interesting and that they stimulate you to undertake further reading and support you to reflect on your own decision-making skills in practice. The range and types of decisions and dilemmas healthcare practitioners encounter every day in cancer care are exemplified by these case studies, which clearly demonstrate the importance of reflection both in and on action, alongside using the highest quality available contemporary evidence to support decisions. We hope that the cases have encouraged you to think beyond the narrow biomedical and clinical determinants of decision-making to consider service users' psychosocial, spiritual, and politico-economic worldviews.

You may have identified several reoccurring themes across the case studies, for example, care planning, person-centred care, consent, assessment, communication and ethical principles, which explicitly demonstrate the application of the '*6 Cs*' – care, compassion, competence, communication, courage, and commitment (NHS England, 2017). The case studies also show how healthcare practitioners' own values and behaviour should be guided by their professional codes of conduct, reminding us of the expected professional conduct and standards of care expected for all of us.

As you encounter dilemmas and decision-making within clinical practice as your career progresses, Table C.1 provides an overview of some decision-making pitfalls which it is wise to be aware of. Interestingly, the more experienced and confident we become, the more biased we tend to become (Jackson, 2021). For instance, if we have encountered something similar previously, we are more likely to draw comparisons the next time. Although this means that exposure to clinical practice brings valuable clinical judgement, it may also mean we may take shortcuts with our decision-making (Jackson, 2021). As mentioned in the introduction, we bring our own world view and sometimes the influences of our home lives to situations, which at times can cloud our judgement. Always use the team around you when feasible to guard against any unconscious bias (Oxtoby, 2020).

In conclusion, working in a caring role can be profoundly rewarding, as being alongside others when they are at their most vulnerable and scared is both a privilege and incredibly fulfilling. When you began your career in healthcare, you may have had high expectations of yourself and given little thought to the impact of this type of work on your daily life, either physically or emotionally. However, in a real-world clinical situation, it can be difficult at times, and the most important thing to remember is to give yourself permission to look after yourself and have some self-compassion. Take time to support and reassure your work colleagues, and do not hesitate to reach out for support when you need it. Keep alert to signs of

DOI: 10.4324/9781003651758-19

Anchoring bias	being overly reliant on the first piece of information
Clustering illusion	tendency to see patterns in random events
Blind spot bias	not noticing either cognitive or motivational bias in ourselves
Ostrich effect	ignoring dangerous or negative information
Resource bias	decisions actively influenced by availability of resources
Availability heuristic	overestimating the importance of available information
Confirmation bias	listening only to information which confirms our preconceptions
Recency bias	weighting latest information more heavily than previous evidence
Over-optimism	too confident in our decision and taking greater risks
Repetition bias	tendency to attach weight to the most repeated story
Similarity bias	favouring the information presented by people who are 'like us'
Conservatism bias	favouring prior evidence over up-to-date information
Group think bias	safety in numbers makes people reluctant to appear to think differently from the group
Sunk-costs bias	following through on a course of action because we previously invested in it
Authority bias	basing decisions on the attributes and opinions of an authority figure and putting personal opinion on hold

Table C.1 Decision pitfalls

Source: Jackson (2021).

compassion fatigue, stress, or burnout, and take proactive steps to avoid these in the first place. See further reading for sources of advice, support, and where to get help. Finally, remember that when you feel both physically and mentally well, you can provide the highest quality services and the most compassionate experience for those in your care.

Further reading

Cavell Nurses Trust (2022) *Help and advice.* https://cavellnursestrust.org (Accessed 19th December 2022).

NHS England (2021) *Professional Nurse Advocate Programme.* https://www.england.nhs.uk/nursingmidwifery/delivering-the-nhs-ltp/professional-nurse-advocate/ (Accessed 5th January 2023).

NMC (2020) *Mental health and wellbeing.* nmc.org.uk (Accessed 19th December 2022).

Nurse Lifeline: *Supporting Mental Health and Emotional Wellbeing.* https://www.nurselifeline.org.uk (Accessed 4th January 2023).

Royal College of Nursing (2015) *Stress and you: A guide for nursing staff.* rcn.org.uk (Accessed 20th December 2022).

Royal College of Nursing (2019) *Beating burn out.* rcn.org.uk (Accessed 5th January 2023).

Royal College of Nursing Counselling Service. https://www.rcn.org.uk/Get-Help/Member-support-services (Accessed 30th June 2025)

References

Jackson, A. (2021) *Dilemmas and Decision Making in Social Work.* St. Albans, Critical Publishing.

NHS England (2017) *Introducing the 6 C's.* https://www.england.nhs.uk (Accessed 5th January 2023).

Oxtoby, K. (2020) How unconscious bias can discriminate against patients and affect their care. *British Medical Journal*, 371. https://doi.org/10.1136/bmj.m4152

Index

For Product Safety Concerns and Information please contact our EU
representative GPSR@taylorandfrancis.com
Taylor & Francis Verlag GmbH, Kaufingerstraße 24, 80331 München, Germany

www.ingramcontent.com/pod-product-compliance
Lightning Source LLC
Chambersburg PA
CBHW061241220326
41599CB00028B/5500